EVEN GOURMANDS
HAVE TO DIET

THE TRAVELING GOURMAND SERIES

1. *The Gluten-Free Way: My Way*, by William Maltese & Adrienne Z. Milligan
2. *Back of the Boat Gourmet Cooking: Afloat—Pool-Side—Backyard*, by Bonnie Clark & William Maltese
3. *William Maltese's Wine Taster's Diary: Spokane/Pullman Washington Wine Region*, by William Maltese
4. *In Search of the Perfect Pinot G! Australia's Mornington Peninsula: William Maltese's Wine Taster's Guide #2*, by A. B. Gayle & William Maltese
5. *Whole Wheat for Food Storage: Recipes for Unground Wheat*, by Michael R. Collings & Judith Collings
6. *Even Gourmands Have to Diet: It's Just Food, People!*, by Bonnie Clark and William Maltese

EVEN GOURMANDS HAVE TO DIET

IT'S JUST FOOD, PEOPLE!
THE TRAVELING GOURMAND
BOOK SIX

BONNIE CLARK &

WILLIAM MALTESE

THE BORGO PRESS
MMXI

EVEN GOURMANDS HAVE TO DIET

Copyright © 2011 by Bonnie Clark and
William Maltese
Cover by Deana C. Jamroz

FIRST EDITION

Published by Wildside Press LLC

www.wildsidebooks.com

DEDICATION

BONNIE—

For my husband, **Bruce**, without whom this book wouldn't have been possible. A man who loves to eat, his joining me in a dieting regimen initially didn't seem possible. Then, I just began fixing meals for us that were reduced in calories and proportions, even found a shake which he loved for its taste and convenience. Without his even realizing it, at least at first, he became part of "our" diet plan. Certainly, as my official taster, in making recipes more diet-friendly, he was invaluable.

WILLIAM—

I'll join Bonnie in dedicating this book to **Bruce** who, although not given joint author credit, probably deserves it.

CONTENTS

DISCLAIMER 9
XOÇAI®...OR NAY 10
BONNIE 12
THE "BIG" WHY? 23
WILLIAM 42
CHECK WITH YOUR DOCTOR 46
WHAT WORKS FOR US 47
THINK AGAIN 48
THE DEVIL IS IN THE FOOD 50
IT'S JUST FOOD, PEOPLE! 52
SNACKS 55
ENERGY DRINKS, POP, AND CANDY 62
EXERCISE 64
OUR/YOUR JOURNAL 70
WEIGHING IN 72
OUR DIET REGIME 73
WATER 76

CALORIE COUNTS	78
ORAC	80
SHAKES	85
FOOD GROUPS AND RECIPES	88
RECIPES	91
SOUPS	92
SALAD	99
SALAD DRESSINGS	101
VINEGAR	109
VEGETABLES	111
FISH AND SEAFOOD	125
DAIRY	136
FOWL	138
SAUCES	147
PASTAS	151
BREADS	155
DESSERTS	158
WINES	160
RECIPE INDEX	162
ABOUT THE AUTHORS	164

DISCLAIMER

All organizations, businesses, and product names mentioned in this book are the property of those individual organizations and businesses. In this day and age of the internet, when so many organizations, businesses, and products are so often mentioned without their attending trademark designates ™ or ®, it's difficult to know when or if to provide these indicators. Even specific searches of U.S. Trademark Department files can often be confusing. So, more often than not, the authors have erred on the side of inclusion, rather than exclusion. If mistakes have been made, every attempt will be made to assure they're corrected in subsequent editions.

XOÇAI®...OR NAY

Throughout this book are references to MXI Corporation products, Xoçai® the healthy chocolate. Each time this occurs, it should be assumed these are nothing more than suggestions that can be substituted with any similar products (after carefully reading labels) provided by some other company. That the authors have given MXI's Xoçai® the healthy chocolate prominence is only because those products are what the authors personally used/use, and their listing all available and viable alternatives would have proved too labor intensive, seen some left out, and, possibly, have resulted in confusion.

Granted, the authors are such enthusiasts that they've each become an official distributor of Xoçai® the healthy chocolate (Maltese's reason admittedly more to obtain it for his own consumption at wholesale prices), but MXI is neither an official sponsor of this book, nor has it had any official say, affiliation, or participation, in the book's writing and/or publication. All of the authors' claims and statements, regarding Xoçai® the healthy chocolate, are entirely their personal observations and opinions, and not those of MXI.

For those interested in learning more about Xoçai® the healthy chocolate, visit either Bonnie or William's official distribution web-sites at:

http://www.richesinchocolate.com
http://www.mxi.myvoffice.com/williammaltese

BONNIE

While this book *does* include some recipes of William and my favorite gourmet dishes that we've incorporated in our respective regimens to stay thin and healthy, it's more than *just* a recipe book, in that it chronicles my personal story of getting fat, how I struggled with my fatness, and how I—finally—found the path to healthy thinness while being able to eat well. It's about all of the helpful tips and techniques I've personally acquired on my difficult journey.

Just because "gourmet" and "gourmand" appear frequently, our recipes aren't expensive, difficult, or complicated. In fact, to us, "gourmet" mainly just means "special."

Bon Appétit!

On Dieting

The reason I could never stay on a diet was because I really didn't want to. There, I said it. I always let myself get in my own way. Had I wanted to stay the course, I would have. I just, each time, had my bag of tricks (excuses) to justify why I couldn't. These included everything from…no time for proper planning…

to…I've a medical problem so I can't really diet, period. Sound familiar?

A Serial Dieter

From the get-go, I'll tell you I'm *not* (nor is William) a doctor of any kind. Not a scientist. Not a nutritionist. Not a single "letter" behind my/our names. I *was* a Serial Dieter. If there's a diet out there, I've probably been on it...low carb; no carb; low fat; no fat; low calorie; high protein; low protein; small portions; starvation; binge; cabbage soup; lemonade with cayenne pepper; food one day, only liquid the next; grapefruit and eggs; fat-flushing diet; Weight Watchers®; Jenny Craig®; Nutrisystem®…. Got the idea? Seldom skinny. Almost always fat. And I do *mean* fat. I'm not going to try and pretty that word up, in that fat is *fat* is Fat is FAT.

All diets work for some people, or those diets wouldn't still be around. And they all usually, at least for awhile, worked for me; but, if the diets really *were* the secrets to a healthy and thin me that they all purported to be, why did I need to keep trying new ones? Why did each and every one of them eventually quit working? What happened? Why did I fall off the wagon, so to speak?

Weight loss is a billion-dollar-a year-industry, to which I have made more than my fair share of contributions.

Even when I lost the weight I wanted to lose, I only ended up, in the end, thinking, "Great. Now, I can get back to eating all those foods I couldn't have on that dang diet." Sometimes, my sole goal was to lose weight just so I *could* eat those foods—again—in the same quantities that made me fat in the first place.

When William and I, with the help of my husband, Bruce (our official grill-master and food-tester), wrote our best-selling cookbook, BACK OF THE BOAT GOURMET COOKING, for the Borgo Press "The Traveling Gourmand" series, the necessary testing, and tasting of our recipes, mandatory before publication, provided me with yet another excuse to overeat. I reasoned that since our food was, for the most part, "healthy", then, it had to be good for me, purposely overlooking the obvious reality that, especially in dieting, there can be too much of even a good thing. Such rationalizations, and such overlooking, were more reasons I didn't last very long on any diet—or even on combinations there of, although I did try.

Mother Dearest

Every diet I was ever on had one thing in common. DEPRIVATION. No matter how much I ate—WOW!—five cups of broccoli—I still felt hungry for *something* I couldn't have and which was a definite no-no on whatever diet I was on.

Who can keep up, forever, on diets with so many *couldn't* and *shouldn't*, *can't* and *don't*? Apparently, not I, who just seemed doomed to be forever fat, unable to help myself in always wanting to eat whatever I was thinking about eating at any one time. I hated being deprived. It brought back childhood memories of my parents telling me I couldn't do *this,* or couldn't *have that.* I don't remember what it was I may have wanted to do, or have, as a kid, but I *do still* remember *not* getting to do or have it. Possibly, what I wanted wasn't good for me. No matter! Same with the food I wanted during dieting. I knew ooey-gooey things weren't good for me. I knew that any high-piled plate of "whatever" wasn't going to be good for me, either. Knowing seldom kept me from wanting and, eventually, eating.

The *Catch-22* was always that, after I ended up eating whatever...giving in to the temptation and loving each and every bite of it...I, then, beat myself up for having been so weak as to have succumbed to eating something so good-tasting but so bad for me. Forever, I chided myself for lack of will power.

My Mother, thinking, mistakenly, that she could shame me into losing the 50-plus pounds I gained while pregnant, *pregnancy the ultimate excuse for eating,* would go to second-hand stores to get me clothes, because she didn't want "to *waste* a lot of money on fat clothes"; her words, not mine. She'd come back with clothes with the biggest arm holes she could find. She would hold these up for me and say, "Do you think these sleeves are big enough for *your* arms, Bonnie?" Bless her little pea-pickin' heart. I suppose she meant well, but boy, how that hurt—and the memory of it still does. Did it make me lose weight? NO. Quite to the contrary, it usually sent me into an eating frenzy. Did you ever do that? Try to drown your hurt in a big piece of chocolate cake, or in a big bag of chips and a big bowl of dip, or in a big carton of ice cream—washing all of that down with your tears? Right now, just thinking about it, has me teary-eyed because of how absolutely hopeless I felt.

Even if I managed, somehow, to muster some self-control, self-disciple, and/or willpower, for however long, it was only momentary. Mainly, it was the forever "battle of the bulge". Was I destined to be hopelessly fighting non-stop not to be *fat,* Fat, FAT.

Talking to Myself

I became an expert at self-talk. Not the good kind, either. I would start by mentally kicking myself; firstly, because I *was* that fat; secondly, because I somehow *deserved* to be that fat.

Deserved to be fat? Whatever does that mean? Why are so many of us so against ourselves? Maybe, in the end, it's just because we really can't blame anyone but ourselves…not even our mothers.

Sad but true!

Look around. Aren't there thin and healthy people out there? There are a lot of them. Why do they "deserve" to be thin and not us? Why did I think they could be thin and healthy, and I could not? I thought they were "different" from me, but the only difference was that they were willing to eat healthy and to exercise, where I—at some point— was not. When I realized that important fact, I had to adjust my thinking big time and only blame myself.

I had a chubby friend who I wrongly admired,

because she *seemed* so comfortable in her own fat-filled skin. She wore sleeveless dresses and sleeveless tops. I would never have done that. I was way too self-conscious to even have one sleeveless "anything" in my wardrobe. If I'd ever worn such a thing, even under a jacket, and, for whatever the reason had had to remove my jacket, I would have died from the embarrassment of anyone seeing my big fat arms. No matter that my wearing only long sleeves made me horribly uncomfortable in summer.

We can think we don't care about being fat, but, inside, we really do. Even my friend, seemingly so self-confident, one day, quite unexpectedly (at least to me) dissolved into a puddle of confessed insecurity because of her weight. I was shocked, in that I had so long looked up to her as the epitome of "fat and happy". My reasoning had always been…If *she* can be that way, then, dang, *I* can be fat and happy, too. We tell ourselves all sorts of lies, and make all sorts of rationalizations, to make ourselves feel better about ourselves.

I'm not saying it's not okay to feel fine about yourself if you're plus-size. If you're content, are healthy, feel good, have lots of energy, and can do everything you want to do, then good for you. However, if it's all a charade, just another cover-up excuse for having let yourself go, and for thinking you are unable to do anything about it, then shame on you.

Pie in the Sky

Apparently, obesity is now epidemic. Government studies put 67% of our population in the fat-zone, and that percentage has been projected to increase by 2% every year. By my calculation, in about fifteen years, we're all scheduled to explode.

How many of our children, and our children's children, have been raised on macaroni and cheese from that little blue box? How much nutrition in those toaster-pastries we give our children for breakfast, fooling ourselves into thinking at least our kids are getting a breakfast? How many breaded mystery-chicken chunks, deep-fried and dipped in mystery sauce, have we all eaten, again trying to fool ourselves that chicken is healthier than, say, hamburger? Do many of us even know, anymore, what a fresh vegetable is or even looks like? Do our children know?

I would venture that if you're reading this book, you are, like I was, a Serial Dieter, still not happy about your size. You've tried diets, and, although, they've all failed you, in one way or another, you're not ready to give up—not yet, anyway. Maybe, just maybe, this diet just might be "the" one that will work for you. Maybe, just maybe, the game plan advocated in this book, complete with tasty gourmet diet recipes, *will* be the one that performs the magic that let's you dismount, slim and trim, from that seemingly never-ending serial-dieter's merry-go-round ride.

Metamorphosis? Not!

What do you have to show for all those diets undergone? I only know, I was left with the same "thunder" thighs, belly bulge, flabby arms, and, more than once, with even an increased shoe size (if you can believe!). Nothing changed, at least for long, after my having starved to be free of that pound or two that was soon gained back, along with additional fat.

Did/do you, like I, try to fool yourself into believing that if you lost 2 or 3 pounds, and you gained back 3, 4, or 5, you *really* gained *only* 2 pounds, 3 pounds, or whatever? Now, I do agree that 2, 3, or even a 5 pound gain isn't too bad. But, add that to the weight you already needed to lose, and, well….

The "Little" Why?

Why did we put ourselves through all those failed attempts to get thin? For a class reunion? For a wedding? For a spouse? For a Mother/Mother-in-law? For summer, and swimming-suit weather, on the horizon? Whatever the reason, did it work? If so, for how long?

So, we lost some of the flab. Or, maybe, we didn't. I usually did, but it didn't stay off for long. It always found its way back, bringing those new fat "friends" right along with it. Dang!

What was my problem? It couldn't have been that I didn't want Tom Stud-Muffin, from my senior year in high school, to see what he'd missed out on, because I *did* want that, especially after having heard that some of the cheerleaders had let themselves "go". Yes! I would show everyone up who wasn't in shape. Or, was it that I just couldn't take any more of my aunt's patronizing fat remarks at one more family reunion? Maybe, my husband wasn't looking at me as he once had when I was thinner. Oh, how *that* hurts! Maybe, I even caught him looking, or even "chatting up" a "thin woman". Ouch! Of course, I could always tell myself that *he* wasn't the same as he once was, either. Did doing that, though, make me feel any better? Okay, maybe it did, but only for a while.

Why was I so hard on myself? Why are some of us harder than others on ourselves? Do those people who seem not to care about being fat *really* not care, or are they really cringing on the inside, like my friend, at the thought of what others are thinking?

I read all the books with all their psycho-babble about loving myself and my body. And, that worked for a while, too, usually until I put the book down and the next pastry cart rolled by with another one of its beautifully enticing ooey-gooey super-delicious pieces of pure bliss that jumped right into my mouth. Hey, why and how did that happen? Or, if I was dieting with a friend, or with my husband, there was always, the—*wink**wink*—"I'll eat one if you do. He-he." Boy did *that* always seem to make it all right. You know what I mean (that's *not* a question).

How about the *uber*-excuse of my slow metabolism? Obviously, Skinny Sarah got to stuff her face and not gain an ounce, *because she had a faster metabolism* than I did. Why did I only just have to look at a French fry, and my hips went all flabby? And Sarah didn't even profess to care all that much about food, saying, she only "eats when hungry." Imagine that!

Maybe, just maybe, though, my metabolism wasn't and isn't slow. Could it be that all of those thyroid tests I've insisted my doctor perform, over the years (try and blame the thyroid!), weren't necessary? Maybe, just maybe, I was always just eating too much, too fast; my metabolism unable to keep up.

On and off diets, I was always hungry—for something. Oh sure, the diet gurus told me the reason for that was that I was just *thirsty*. My body was trying to say it was dehydrated, not hungry. Just drink a glass of water—a very *large* glass of water—and wah-lah—my hunger would be gone. Yeah, right. Who did they think they were kidding? It might have worked for Skinny Sarah, but what did she know? It sure never worked for me, except for, maybe, a quick minute or two when I drank so much water that I sloshed when I walked—and I *did* try that, more than once—ending up with a persistent gnawing hunger in my gut and a violent need to pee.

They—whoever, *they* are—told me I should rate my hunger pangs from 1 to 10; ten equal to my having stuffed myself at Thanksgiving dinner; one equal to my having become so hungry I was tempted to eat my own arm. They told me it was so I could always eat when feeling about "5"; just hungry enough to think I wanted something. Why, then, after stuffing myself so many times at a Thanksgiving dinner table, did I find myself still able to eat more—if just that small piece of Grandma's pumpkin pie; after all, I didn't want to hurt her feelings? Why did I waddle off to bed, after that, moaning and groaning, and swearing not to eat for a week, only to get up in the morning—wah-lah, leftovers!—to start eating all over again?

I could go on and on about this or that failed diet of mine. I could go on and on about my trick-or-treat rationalizations for each and every failed diet. But….

THE "BIG" WHY?

"To be or not to be—that is the question:
Whether 'tis nobler in the mind to suffer
The slings and arrows of outrageous fortune,
Or to take arms against a sea of troubles
And, by opposing, end them."
William Shakespeare

You have probably heard the above quote as many times as I have. But have you ever thought of it with your weight problem in mind? Would you rather *suffer the slings and arrows* of mean and cruel people, or *arm* yourself by opposing them? Or, better yet—realize it's not about them? I was guilty of slinging the most arrows at myself.

I've such a passion on the subject of weight-loss (or lack there of), that it's been a weight—no pun intended—on my heart (as well as on my body) for a very long time; it still is.

Some people gain a little weight, for whatever the cause, diet it off, and that's that. Not I. Why? For some reason, my weight gains all seemed intent upon hanging around to become an integral part of the physical me. Not just as additions to my belly, or my thighs, but as part of the "mental" me. As a result, I became obsessed with losing weight. Of course, the more I dieted and failed at dieting, the more obsessed I became about dieting, and the more I thought about dieting, the more I wanted to eat (and usually did) while dieting.

All of which, I've come to realize, was the result of my "why" for dieting not being nearly "big enough".

Do you remember when Oprah Winfrey lost all that weight the *first* time? You know, those 67 pounds and she came out on stage in that pair of really skinny jeans, looking absolutely fabulous, and pulling that wagon with sixty-seven pounds of REAL FAT on board? From that day forward, however, proud as she was of her weight loss, she started, admittedly, gaining the weight back.

Why? Because, she'd wanted to lose that particular sixty-seven pounds of fat, and she *had* lost it, because she'd had a reason *why*. Namely, she didn't want to show up at an upcoming award's show as fat as she usually did. However, as big a Why as that why had been, it, in the end, didn't turn out to be nearly a BIG enough WHY for her to keep her weight off after the award's show, in question, had come and gone.

I remember another Oprah show where the combined fat losses of her guests were literally megatons. One particular gal had lost a couple hundred pounds of it, all by herself, and still retained all of her anger about how she'd been talked about and treated by other people—men, women, airline personnel, waiters, waitresses, co-workers, even her family and supposed friends—when she'd been fat. She felt everyone had looked down on her, and she had "that" as her Why, in order to show *them* all that she could be as thin as anyone. Was that a BIG enough WHY, though, for her to keep the weight off? I don't know. I can only hope so. It did, though, seem to have been more about *them,* and how *they* felt about *her* fat.

All I know is that I've lost weight for more than one Why in my time. I'm sure you have too.

For instance, I had a nasty, mean-spirited sister-in-law who loved to point out how she thought I looked like I had "put on a few pounds". After my son was born, and I *ha*d put a few pounds, this sister-in-law was particularly mean-spirited and informed me that I was a "disgrace to womanhood". Of course, she was one of those people that I, for some masochistic reason, looked up to, at the time, if just because she seemed to have "it" all together—every hair in place; a house that was immaculate—a yard exquisitely landscaped—clothes always gorgeous and perfectly fitted. Every time she would come *at* me, I would, of course, vow to lose weight. However, if I lost weight, she would, then, tell me I looked "sickly". Eventually, I discovered she was an alcoholic and not nearly as "with it" as I had always supposed. She and her husband moved to another state for many years, and I didn't have to deal with her. When I found out they were moving back, my first reaction was to worry about what she would say about the pounds I'd packed on in her absence. Sure enough, the first thing she said to me was, "My, I see you've gained a few pounds." Well, this time, for some reason, I countered, "Well, some of us eat and some of us *drink*." The look on her face was priceless, and she was never mean to me again. After that turning point, however, what she thought of me was no longer a big enough Why for me to want to diet.

Nor was it a big enough Why whenever summer showed up, with our pool surrounded by our usually large and frequent groups of houseguests. Then, of course, there was all of the time we spent at the lake, on our boat, with suntanned and slim bikini-clad bodies all around. In each scenario, I tried to keep from looking like a beached whale by merely not putting on a swim suit or by not wearing short sleeves. As if either of those really ever worked.

MY "BIG" WHY?

When I experienced a couple of minor strokes, spending a lot of recuperative time as a lump on the couch, mainly depressed, I suddenly had several more good excuses for any weight I gained—and I gained a lot. At the time, my love of "unhealthy" chocolates didn't help things any, in fact only made my weight gain all the more noticeable, especially when I started looking upon chocolates as better friends than those people who had suddenly stopped coming by to visit.

Bruce and I started out each eating *one* very expensive, absolutely decadent, rich chocolate truffle every night, usually after a sizable dinner. We fooled ourselves into thinking just *one* chocolate truffle, apiece, was better for us than each of us eating a big piece of pie, cake, tort, or half a dozen cookies. Before too long, we rationalized each of us having *two* truffles a night, convincing ourselves, once again, that we were doing nothing bad for/to our bodies. Certainly, the chocolate company never said its truffles *weren't* healthy. Its claim was that its chocolate was "the best chocolate". That it was "a wonderful treat". That we "deserved to indulge". All too easy a spiel for us to swallow (pun intended), hook, line, and truffle.

A couple of things, though, pretty much concurrent, ended up providing me with my BIG WHY, as apparently needed for me personally to achieve, finally, some long-run success in dieting.

One, a friend dropped by and suggested that if Bruce and I were going to eat chocolate, we should at least eat the "healthy" chocolate, Xoçai®, which provides far more advantages than the regular "stuff", if just because it's so full of antioxidants. By substituting Xocai® chocolates for the bad, we could still indulge our penchants for decadent, luscious dark chocolate, but eat it in a healthier form.

At first, of course, Bruce and I did a lot of *wink**wink*, as regards any such chocolate claiming to be "good and healthy". We were so used to tricking ourselves into making anything we wanted to eat okay to eat, that we'd decided to believe her pitch line whether it was true or not.

As it turns out, my friend was one-hundred percent right, as far as we're concerned. That doesn't mean that, having since become an official Xoçai® distributor, I'm now going to give you a sales pitch on Xoçai® the healthy chocolate, as a means of making money, via my web-site. I am going to say that Bruce and I personally bear witness to not only having lost weight while eating Xoçai®, but we've kept the lost weight off. Likewise, we drink Xoçai® High Protein, High Antioxidant Meal Replacement Shakes®. All of which are convenient for our busy lives, especially since they're not loaded with refined sugars, sweeteners, fats, caffeine, or other bad stuff that our bodies can't use and shouldn't have. They are dairy-free, gluten-free, diabetic- and vegan-friendly, which are things we've discovered we need to be aware. If you prefer some other shake, protein bar, or diet cookie, that's fine; just read its label, and be sure it's right for you, in that some are loaded with sugars, imitation or real, fats, and other bad-for-you things we can't even pronounce. Most of us get fat by putting junk into our bodies; so, for heaven's-sake, don't.

Two, by way of providing me with a BIG WHY, was my cousin, William Maltese, co-author with me on this book, who appeared one day on my doorstep, after a long absence of traveling the world, and invited me (with the assist of my husband Bruce), to join him in capitalizing upon our combined fondness for boating, grilling, and gourmet food, by writing our first cookbook collaboration, *BACK OF THE BOAT GOURMET COOKING: BOAT, POOLSIDE, AND BACK-YARD.*

Truthfully, in the past, my love of cooking, my love

of food, my love of entertaining and feeding people, were just other big excuses I could always pull out of my bag of tricks to explain any weight gain. This time, though, faced with the sudden necessity of getting "out there" into the public "eye", prompted by William, who insisted I promote "our upcoming book", then promote our "officially published book", by way of signings, reviews, and local photo shoots of our recipes for cuisine magazines, found me less inclined to accept gaining weight while cooking, eating, entertaining, and feeding the people who became our official "food samplers".

NOTE: While recovering from a series of little strokes, the weakness in my right arm made it impossible for me to do much cooking. Having for years spoiled Bruce with homemade meals (he wasn't, in those days, all that handy in the kitchen), we were suddenly eating those fast foods most convenient for him to bring home so that we could eat in private. During that time, we became prime examples of each and every study that pointed to, "Yes, indeed, folks, you *can* get fat on take-out!"

In the process of "becoming" a published, author, I took a closer look at my wardrobe, which I'd been wearing to hide my fat, or, because I pretended it didn't make any difference how I looked because I was fat.

In short, I'd become self-rooted in a self-pitying mode that had allowed me to dress "down" and not look my best when I should have been doing just the opposite.

I did have a hairdresser/friend who, even if I didn't know it, knew I needed a with-it hairdo, to feel better about myself. We've all heard of "bad hair" days, but there are '"bad hair" years, too. Thank you René for guiding me into making that discovery.

I realized I needed a makeup makeover. Although I'd never let anyone see me *without* makeup, I wasn't up-to-date in that department. Just as we shouldn't likely forever wear the same hairdo we did in high school, we likely shouldn't wear the same makeup we did when we were in our teens.

As I looked to others for fashionable ideas, I saw I wasn't the only one who let myself go. At least, I wore makeup; some women didn't, their hair looking anything but stylish. I never did reach the point where I'd think of wearing lounging pajamas outsides of my own home, having noted how many people, men and women, did just that, as well as wore their bedroom *slippers* to malls, stores, and restaurants.

What was it with all those bare, white, ugly legs? Who started that unflattering trend? As low as I felt, I never left the house with bare, white ugly legs on show. Hadn't those women heard of self-tanning products? Besides, as we age, we get these lovely veins, brown spots, and other things I call "barnacles". Self-tanning gels hide these nicely. Get a good brand—no orange! And do something about those ugly, dry, cracked heels! Lotion, lotion, lotion!

Speaking of feet, what is with those ugly rubber

clodhoppers, which come in every color of the rainbow, and some people call shoes? Granted, even I have a pair, bought at a garden supply store, but I only wear them in my garden, never "in public". As for "work" shoes, they should be worn at work, and then left there.

Even when I was unable to wear high heels after my strokes, I bought flat shoe that were gold, silver, and copper: pretty and stylish. With the right shoes, hair, makeup, even a classy purse, I could believe I was on my way to feeling good and feeling pretty. The great thing about doing these types of things, too, was how I could do them and they "fit", no matter what size I was.

Persuaded by William to be out and about to promote our book, I made a conscious effort to dress and look better, thereby feel better. If I was still fat, I was no longer in a self-pitying downward spiral, and actually started digging myself out of the hole in which I'd been.

In fact, William was so impressed by the results of my healthy chocolate regime, combined with our healthy wine-paired gourmet recipes for BACK OF THE BOAT GOURMET COOKING, which had me feeling so damned good and losing weight, he suggested we start substituting Xoçai® in all of our recipes that called for chocolate. Then, he joined me in eating Xoçai®, not as a way for him to lose weight but as a way for him to maintain his present weight and stay healthy in the process.

MY BIG WHY? Got BIGGER

My real epiphany came the moment I realized that I had suddenly become entirely less needful of the approval of others and their congratulatory or consolatory pats on my back which had, likely, more often than not, been less than truly heart-felt anyway.

By way of Whys, things like award's shows come and go (just ask Oprah); summers and school reunions come and go (just ask me). In the end, it merely boils down to no one but me being accountable for my success or failure in dieting, or in anything else...the only person I need please is ME; it doesn't matter what others think. I have to like ME. I have to love ME. I need to care about ME, not *just* by getting thin, but by eating healthy and *being* healthy, both physically and mentally. I underwent a total mind-shift: *positive attitude so much more than just positive thinking.*

I spotted a Macy's woman's clothing ad in the newspaper. The model-in-the-dress had exactly "the look" I wanted to achieve for my new image. So what if the model in the ad was a smaller dress size than I was?

I cut the ad out and pasted it on the front of my refrigerator. Whenever I thought about overeating, or whenever I *thought* I was hungry, I looked at that picture of that model and that dress, and I reminded myself that I was a published author, with a mainstream press, out and about, enjoying myself, thinner than I'd been in years, and I'd eat yet another piece of healthy Xoçai® chocolate instead of junk food. Then, I'd close my eyes and "become" the model in that ad. It didn't even matter that she had dark hair and that I'm strawberry blonde (natural, of course). I just told myself that I was in control. How had I ever come to believe otherwise?

Every morning, before I stepped into the shower, I looked at *that/my* picture. I held it in my mind's-eye as I showered. I *felt* being that thin. As I washed, I *felt* my arms and legs smaller; my hips narrower; my tummy flatter; my thighs, and, oh, my, yes, even my butt so much tinier. I *felt* my hipbones reappear after long years of being missing in action. My hair *felt* silkier, because it and I were so much healthier. I *felt* what it was like to slip that skinny little outfit over my slim, trim, body. Ah, so good! I donned gorgeous slim shoes on my slender, soft, callus-free, perfectly pedicured feet. I became giddy; it was all so good. I didn't let negative thoughts intrude and/or interfere.

I looked in the mirror and said, in my best Barbra Streisand voice,"Hello Gorgeous!"

I carried that feeling with me all day. Sometimes, I might have gotten discouraged, but I just constantly reassured myself as to WHY I remained in control.

I pictured the foods I would eat as always being healthy foods, always tasting good, always providing me with a healthy over-all glow and feeling of well-being and contentment. As soon as a visual of junk food tried to intrude, I shot it down.

At bedtime, I'd look at "my" ad, wash my face more carefully than I once did, brush my teeth more thoroughly than before, take the time to put lotion on, especially my feet, and even do a few stretching exercises.

Once in bed, I kept imagining what it would feel like actually to look like that model, in that dress, in my ad. Mentally, I crawled into that picture and became her, or, better yet, became *me* in that dress at some party. I walked down a grand staircase, all eyes turned in my direction. My eyes meet admiring eyes, and I knew just how good I looked. I smiled; others smiled back. I was all warm and fuzzy as I chatted with friends and associates, laughing and tossing my luxurious hair. At the buffet tables, I chose all the *right* food, because eating healthy had become so very important to me, by way of my WHY; everything tasting better now that I felt so much better about myself. Wow, the evening was full of fun and laughter. I'd drift off to sleep with the huge smile on my face that was still there the next morning.

I took a picture of my ad with my cell-phone camera, in order to have it with me whenever I needed reassurance of that truly big WHY that kept me successfully on my diet. And, yes, there are times, even now, when I have to "call up" that particular picture for the reassurance it still gives me; so far, I can continue William and my gourmet diet/maintenance plan with the stick-to-it-ness I've previously always found lacking.

What I'm talking about, here, is that *feeling* I get, or have, whenever I know everything is right in my world, including how much I weigh. Do I really believe that I have to be super-model skinny? No! In fact, I've never been, or ever likely will be, true model material, but that's okay as long as I'm feeling healthier and more energetic than I ever have. Truly, my pity party, that used to be ongoing, is over, in that I, finally, truly, do like ME.

Don't even think, for even one brief moment, about posting a fat picture of you on the refrigerator. That is *so* negative and detrimental, why would you ever want to concentrate on that? Keep a positive picture of yourself in your mind's-eye. You'll be battling enough negative thoughts, as it is, and you don't need something like that on full view. I speak from painful experience, once having had just such a fat picture of me posted, albeit inside a cupboard door. No one even knew it was there, except for my husband and for me. I would look at it and tell myself how fat I was. How awful I looked. I'd call myself names like Fat Bonnie. That was just a whole lot of negative input that I only now recognize was something I definitely didn't need, have never needed, and, hopefully, will never-ever need again. There's an old saying…where the mind goes, the body follows. In the case of my big-fat picture, I continually reinforced my existing thoughts of myself as Fat Bonnie, and I stayed Fat Bonnie. Of more help, as I've since discovered with the Macy's ad, is some more positive image, on which to focus positive concentration.

I hope you get the idea. It is not just *picturing* you thin—it's actually *feeling* it. I had a WHY. But a WHY is just the beginning. I was literally pushed from the nest (AKA, couch), by William who insisted I get on out into the land of the living. I started, first, by feeling how bad I was going to feel meeting people in the state I felt I was in. I had to push that aside! Too negative! If I concentrated on how fat I was, and how I had let myself go, I would have ended up at a party, alright, but it would have been my own pity party. I had to do this for me and only for me. You see my WHY started with what I perceived people would think of me, rather than asking myself how that made *me feel*; how I wanted them to think of me, rather than asking myself how that made *me feel*; until I finally figured out it came down to how *I felt* about *me,* not about how they felt about me. If others thought I was fat, or if I thought others thought I was fat, it was because I *was* fat. It was time I either "got over it", and became fat and happy, or took sole responsibility for getting healthy and losing the extra baggage—literally.

We've one of those scales with ounces on it. It used to be that if I lost only a few ounces a day, or a week, when I so yearned to lose so much more, I was sent running to drown my sorrow in another tub of ice cream hidden in the very back of the freezer, specifically kept there to feed just such frustrations. Now, I know that I should constantly celebrate whatever my weight loss, large or however small. Funny how, when the scale said, let's say, 130.6 on Tuesday morning, and 130 on Wednesday, I felt I hadn't lost anything when, in actuality, I had lost 6 ounces. However, if the scale said 130.5 on Tuesday morning and 129.9 on Wednesday, I would jump for joy, because, in my mind, I had lost a whole pound, when I'd still only lost 6 ounces. When

I let this reality set in, I started celebrating any loss of ounces, and this helped everything else start to fall into place.

Some days, your clothes may feel tight, not because of a weight gain but only because of bloating. Bloating is nothing more than a lot of hot air, if you know what I mean, and it doesn't show up on the scale. So don't obsess about it, because it will pass (pun intended).

Remember—Get Over It!

> *"We must all suffer from one of two pains: the pain of discipline, or the pain of regret. The difference is that discipline weighs ounces, while regret weighs tons."*
> —Jim Rohn

Quit using whatever your excuses for not doing what you know you *should* be doing—and for what you're doing that you know is wrong for you to be doing, although you keep on doing them. Realize how much better off you'll be when and if you give up all of your so-old-as-to-be-tread-worn excuses.

Start thinking of yourself as naturally thin, and naturally healthy, right here and now. Don't just think it, visualize it, most importantly *feel* it. Don't even wait until you finish reading this book…or until you make resolutions at the beginning of some new year… or a week from Monday…or sometime when you figure you may have the time. After all, why are you waiting? Why aren't you starting right now? Why do you keep constantly playing that same old fat-movie in your head? You know the one. Certainly, I do, in that it's likely a version of the very same one I played and replayed, until I became so comfortable with it, even though it was simultaneously so much my very own personal horror flick, that it was quite easy for me to keep it running constantly while I kept on beating myself up for having no discipline to switch it off, or switch off what was actually the cause of my weight gains. My movie starred my fat. Its audience of one—me—joked about it, cried about it, thought about it, worried about it, obsessed over it, until I finally managed to put an entirely new, and far more positive, reel on the projector. Better yet, I wrote an entirely different script. Why not? We all can, each and every one of us, write whatever the part we play in our own lives, if just because they're our lives to write and live!

In fact, with my new positive movie suddenly running in my mind, my living it, breathing it, feeling it, I was always taken aback when catching a reflection of myself that indicated I wasn't yet as thin and gorgeous as I thought I was. It wasn't that I didn't look better than I did, since I was, after all, taking far much better care of myself than I had been, but it was so strange seeing a fatter person, in reflection, that wasn't how I'd come to perceive the real me.

Pity Party Over

No one is ever really a sure-show at a pity party except the person throwing it. So, don't waste even one more day of your life throwing yourself this kind of to-do. Just STOP IT! Continuing isn't going to do you any good, only keep you miserable, or make you even more so, and, possibly, every one around you. That kind of thinking steals your peace of mind, your joy, and your happiness.

I was smart enough to figure out that this kind of negative activity made me truly miserable. Oh, I wanted to be thinner, healthier, have more energy, but, oh, how I wallowed in self-pity—and ate. By learning to focus on my WHY— how it would feel to be that picture of the svelte model—me—in that perfect 'look'—mine—I got over my pity-parties, and you should and can, too.

How silly it is, after all, to let anything but our positive thoughts control us. Is it easy to break that habit? No! That doesn't mean we *can't* break it. With each pound—or ounce—or partial ounce—lost, it becomes easier to shed the control bad food has over us, as William, Bruce, and I can bear personal witness.

Oh, there are plenty of obstacles along the way—parties, holidays, weddings, lunches with "the guys/gals", doughnuts in the conference rooms, the insistence of your kids that they "want ice cream"…even as thin as William is, he overindulged in some very unhealthy, downright bad foods, while his mother was dying… but we need merely chose *NOW* as our moment. In one year, anyone's life can be truly different; anyone can look better, feel better, be thinner, healthier, and have loads more energy. Where will your life be in a year?

Better? Worse? Thinner? Fatter? The same? Happier? More confident? More miserable? Healthier? Will you be sick? Rundown? Unhealthy? Wishing you had made better choices? Glad you made the right choices?

In the end, you can't *think* yourself thin; you must *feel* your way thin. You don't have to *be* thin to *feel* thin, either. It's all about how thin you *believe* you are, *can* be, *expect* to be, *feel* you are. You just need a mindshift. Start acting like a thin person; after all, you are, now, feeling like a thin and healthy person. There may be people, friends, a spouse, and relatives, maybe even you, who laugh, joke, or make fun of this idea. If you aren't going to stay forever in a fat rut, though, you need to live your own life.

Once, I heard someone say she couldn't go on a diet because she had "way too much weight to lose and it would take *way too long* to lose it." HUH? Whether you have five pounds, or 500 pounds, to lose, *you* have to start, somewhere, sometime. So, make that start today!

> *"The act of taking the first step is what separates the winners from the losers."*
> —Brian Tracy

No excuses. Just do it. If you weren't ready to start, you likely wouldn't be reading this book. So, quit pulling out all of those *unrealistic* rationalizations from your bag of tricks. In fact, throw that damned bag out, once and for all. I mean it. If you procrastinate, and merely put it on some shelf, even way back in your closet, like some cherished keepsake, it'll be way too handy the next time you feel a need to pull out of your diet, and it will come back to haunt you. Right this minute, substitute a positive BIG WHY instead.

WILLIAM

Yes, Virginia, it IS true! Many professional chefs you see ARE, indeed, overweight, chubby, fat, even downright obese. Undoubtedly it has something to do with the mantra of their profession: "Never serve anything you haven't tasted!" Sampling this, sampling that, tasting this, tasting that, CAN, and WILL, put on the pounds.

Nor are others, in professions connected with cooking, immune from weight gain. Food critics CAN and DO gain weight from all of those restaurant visits, during which they're sucked into eating more than they should by rationalizing that their readers are interested in hearing more about the menu of a bistro than the fact it includes delicious diet carrot cake.

Certainly, Bonnie and I…faced as we are, and as we have been in the past, with preparing delicious meals, eating them, and reporting on them (our co-written *BACK OF THE BOAT GOURMET COOKING* comes most immediately to mind)…have had to, and still have to, pay particular attention to the results of all our eating, especially Bonnie who has faced a lifetime of battling weight and image problems.

I have to confess, from the start, that my weight and image problems, from an early age, have been more based upon my long having felt myself too thin, even downright skinny. ["You bugger!" Bonnie says.] I spent a good deal of my youth attempting to *gain* weight by indulging in junk-food binges, chug-a-lugs of innumerable banana milkshakes, and chow-downs on candies, and/or anything else that I hoped would somehow catapult me from skeletal toward that more aesthetically ideal male anatomical perfection provided, in my opinion, by Greco-Roman sculpture. I spent hours performing all of the exercises laid out for me by Charles Atlas, in his muscle-building regime intended to keep me from being one of those skinny kids getting sand kicked in my face by better-built and weightier young men; alas, all to little avail. To my dismay, I remained relatively thin through childhood, adolescence, young manhood, and well into middle-age, all the while little consoled by people who kept telling me, "Enjoy being thin, while you can, because you won't be thin forever." Or, "You can never be too thin or too rich!"

About the time my mother began to die of ovarian cancer, and I stepped in as her sole caregiver...my concern focused more for her all-around health than on assuring that I was eating and exercising properly... my body metabolism finally decided to slow down, and, I, finally, at long last, began putting on weight, albeit in all of the wrong places, to the point where my doctor warned me that I would be of little help in providing for my mother if my own health went down the tube. He pointed direly at my high blood pressure and dangerously high blood-glucose levels (the latter of particular concern because of a history of Diabetes II in my family), as harbingers of bad things to come.

It was only after my mother died, however, when I was actually trying to find one of my several black suits to fit me for her funeral, and not succeeding in fastening the waist of any of their trousers without the help of a safety pin, that I finally took my doctor's advice to lose weight, and, in the process, discovered, for the first time, the difficulties of dieting heard from other people, including Bonnie.

These days, involved as I am in a whole series of ongoing "The Traveling Gourmand" wine- and cookbooks for Wildside/Borgo Press, and, thereby, faced, daily, with the temptation of delicious food and drink, as well as their accompanying calories, I was extremely interested when my fellow gourmands and wine enthusiasts, Bonnie and Bruce Clark, had, at long last, after years of trying, come to believe they had FINALLY found a system of dieting that worked for them.

Seeing how they had, sure enough, stumbled upon a plan, wherein they not only enjoyed gourmet food and fine wine, but still lost weight, found me soon determined to incorporate more and more of what they were doing into my own weight-maintenance regimen. As they predicted, I found it an ideal way of staying thin, feeling healthy, and managing to keep all-important gourmet food and fine wine as major parts of my lifestyle.

In result, Bonnie and I have teamed up, once again, this time around, to write this book based upon her, Bruce, and my, successful dieting that includes some of our gourmet maintaining-our-diet recipes. We believe our success should be shared, especially as regards to Bonnie's often poignant struggles with weight loss and self imagine that likely mirror the same plights of so many others who deserve thin and happy endings.

For anyone needing a handbook to help you either lose weight, or help you maintain an ideal weight, our book, hopefully, will be of some assist, as well as provide recipes for some accompanying fine gourmet-diet dining.

CHECK WITH YOUR DOCTOR

We don't know your medical history or your health problems. We DO know you need to ask your doctor about your personal health issues before going on *any* diet or exercise program. It's "the" most important thing you can do for yourself. Too many of us think we can skip this step. DON'T.

WHAT WORKS FOR US

We're not going to provide a lot of scientific mumbo-jumbo, in that there are plenty of books and websites, out there, that'll give you that—and we recommend you go to them for it. We're just going to tell you what, diet-wise gourmet, and exercise-wise, works for us.

Overweight since high school, Bonnie's husband, Bruce, was well over 200 pounds when he married. What with jobs, kids, and life, the Clarks both gained weight over the years; Bruce ballooned to an all-time high of over 350 pounds. He's not sure just how far over, because his scales only went to 350 pounds at the time. Don't expect Bonnie to provide *her* all-time high, though, because she'd rather tell you her age, and we all know how a lady hardly *ever* tells her age. Now, though, they're both well on their ways to being forever thin, with the help of Xoçai® chocolate, and with this book's supplemental gourmet-diet recipes devised by William and Bonnie, and taste-tested by Bruce, to prove no one has to starve while getting fit, trim, and healthy.

THINK AGAIN

We know you're thinking, even as you read this, that you simply don't really have the kind of money needed to buy the ingredients for "gourmet" food, let alone find the time or energy to follow some time-consuming gourmet recipe.

If so, you can stop any such thinking, because we know all about those times you've not complained about money, time, and energy spent when you whipped up that batch of chocolate-chip cookies just so you could eat the dough…or you headed off in your car to the drive-up window of some never-cheap fast-food joint. While we've come up with some recipes and tips for some mighty tasty food, we've tried to keep the costs down, and the preparations easy.

Our book's chocolate regimen and gourmet-meal recipes have had the most wonderful snowball effect for us. As we eat better—as you can—including Xoçai® chocolate (if that's the route you chose—or not), and as you begin eating the food of our tasty gourmet-diet tips and recipes, and add a little exercise to your daily routine, you, like us, will start to feel better and better, too. We lost weight. We have more energy. So will you. The more energy we have, the more active we become. This will happen to you. The more active we've become, the more weight we've lost. You'll lose more, too. The more weight we've lost, the more we've come to prefer foods good for us. As will you. No more junk food, like fries, chips, sugary candy bars, or Twinkies®. Suddenly, healthy food definitely tastes better.

THE DEVIL IS IN THE FOOD

We truly believe the Devil is wreaking havoc with a lot of people's health. Take the fast-food industry. Satan isn't necessarily that freckled-face kid physically flipping burgers, or taking our orders, but he IS there. Who else would think of super-sizing everything? We just saw an ad for a double-cheese burger made with two mystery meat patties, melted mystery cheese, all sandwiched between TWO *toasted cheese sandwiches* (Yes, we *did* say *sandwiches*!). Oh, we're sure there are those of us eating just such as that and rationalizing why, but wishing we had more control, and, likely, falling asleep in our overstuffed recliners, with beers in our hand, more and more often, each night, these days.

In comparison, whenever we've had a sudden craving for something nutritious, like an apple or even some oatmeal, for instance, haven't we, after the eating, felt exceptionally good? That was our body telling us the right thing to do. Listen to it, because it really does, if given the chance to prove it, know what we really want and need.

How about the time we went out with the "girls" or the "guys" for lunch, ate "healthy", and felt rejuvenated for all the rest of the afternoon, compared with when we went out with them and ate junk food?

Keep thinking about eating healthy versus overindulging on big fat burgers, double or otherwise, or on big fat sandwiches loaded with cheese and mayo, or even on salads drenched in fat-laden dressing and cheese. Believe us when we tell you that you'll feel better, and find gone all slow-motion sluggishness and brain-fog by eating healthy.

Certainly, don't forget that vegetables (more about them, later), are one of the most important food groups in any healthy diet. We've always eaten them, although for years we ate mostly canned, over-cooked ones, with no nutrients left in them. Once we started eating vegetables raw, or that are prepared in healthy ways, we were amazed at just how good they taste. And without a large pat of butter or dripping in dressing, either. A squeeze of lemon or lime will brighten the flavor of vegetables like asparagus or broccoli.

IT'S JUST FOOD, PEOPLE!

You are the master of your food, not vice versa. For Pete's sake, don't let food lord over you. Don't get all overwhelmed by it; just start making the right choices.

Bonnie used to "say" she wanted to be thin, but her "actions" regarding her food choices said otherwise. She just didn't trust her better judgment enough to know she *would*—not just *could*—make the right food choices. She didn't trust herself, enough, where food was concerned, each and every time she started on a new diet. What with her continually wrong food selections, so many of her diets failed that she, as well as others, doubted she'd ever make *any* diet work, which only caused her to distrust even more her ability to pick the right foods.

This is why she was always searching for and trying every diet that came along. She wanted someone to tell her exactly what to eat—and in some cases, when to eat it.

There are all kinds of diets out there, but we can almost guarantee more often than not, you're going to feel deprived in some way, on most of them. But a diet, such as ours, where *you* make the choices, instead of being told what to eat…and *you* choose healthy foods and portion sizes…will see you feeling less deprived. You just have to learn to trust yourself to make those right decisions.

Once, our schedules were full of things to do for everyone but US. Weren't we important? Aren't *you* important? Don't we all deserve some time for ourselves—even if only fifteen minutes, here, or ten minutes, there, to plan, exercise, meditate on our *Why, BIG WHY, BIGGER WHY* to shop the right foods? Although we've always had to go to the grocery store, anyway, and, usually made lists, were those the right choices on that list for our families and for us? If not, why not, since the internet, our computers hooked into it, made it so easy for us to plan truly nutritious meals and snacks?

Finally, though, we set aside those few minutes a day, just for us, to sit quietly and get our thoughts together—yes, even figure out the right foods—and why we'd previously not been paying attention to the simplest rules for right selection, including buying organic.

Such basics, as buying organic, whenever possible, have finally dawned on us, as well as the obviousness of how the less chemical- and toxin-riddled "junk" we put into our bodies, the better we are, the better we feel, and, yes, the better (and less) we want to eat.

Likely, our poor bodies, in the past, had so much trouble trying to figure out the weird chemicals, and additives, with which we were always feeding them that they merely got more and more worn out from continually wrapping up all of that poison in fat: that is how our bodies protect us from toxins we try to digest. Then, our bodies deposit this toxic fat mostly around our bellies, and to our thighs, and to our…yes…rear-ends.

Beware of thinking organic is *too* expensive. Admittedly, it is a bit high-priced, right now, likely always to cost more than its non-organic counterparts, but, when and if fed these foods, free of chemicals and toxins, our bodies achieve a healthy balance that sees us eating less. No longer finding it necessary to eat a whole carton of non-organic berries at a sitting, we're suddenly content to sprinkle merely a few organic berries on our salads, on our cereals, or in our smoothies. Certainly, if you can't pronounce an ingredient on a label, should you risk eating it or feeding it to your family?

Having finally had such a food epiphany doesn't mean forgetting snacks. Instead, access snacks that are as healthy as their counterparts are unhealthy. In our opinions, healthy snacks can be just as important, if not more so, than our selection of healthy food for healthy meals. Sometimes, with our busy schedules, snacks are really all we have time for; therefore, taking the time to plan ahead for healthy ones takes away all our previous excuses for grabbing "unhealthy" ones on the fly. It's time to keep failure always off our tables.

SNACKS

Peanut or almond butters make some great good-tasting snacks. *Always* check labels, because calorie content varies widely, from one brand to another, some having way too much sugar than should be included in our diets. Smooth these butters within the troughs of individual celery sticks—celery a "free food" of which we can eat all we want, without guilt—in order to benefit from the vegetable's fiber. Of course, *always* keep calorie counts on snacks.

At first, we assumed making our own healthy snacks would be horribly expensive, but we were surprised to learn just how inexpensive making them is compared to the cost of the unhealthy snacks we'd been eating. When ground turkey was $3 a pound, and we quartered that for four 4-oz patties (or five 3-oz patties), it only cost us about 75 cents, or less, per snack. And those snacks offered us the high protein our bodies needed to keep us from feeling hungry immediately after snacking. Also, it kept us from getting that late-morning or late-afternoon let-down feeling that, before, had us reaching for something unhealthy.

Does this mean that we never-ever indulge in a not-so-healthy? Absolutely not! We just remember that eating one of something never gives us permission to eat the whole batch—or even 2, 3, or 4. If we desperately crave a cookie, we eat ONE, which it IS possible to do—believe me— if we just remember that we, not the remaining cookies, are the ones in control.

NOTE: By the time this book hits the stands Xocai® should have replaced its Protein Bars with its High Protein, High Fiber, High Antioxidant Diet Cookies® on the market that will be another convenient and healthy snack to keep in our cars, purses, or desk drawers.

Whenever we each drink a shake for breakfast, and one for lunch, with a couple of high-protein snacks or Xocai® chocolate pieces budgeted into the course of each day, concluded by a light dinner, in the evening, we lose weight and/or inches. What's more, we're usually not hungry; in fact, we often have trouble eating our full daily calorie allotments.

Best of all, one of the nutrients in cacao seems capable of doing something to our fat cells, especially around our middles, that shrinks them; hence, often, we lose inches in those often-so-hard-to shrink tummy regions.

As we've said before, planning our snacks is just as important as planning our meals. Most of our snacking is from habit rather than from hunger. By eating high-protein snacks, we find we don't have quite as voracious 3 P.M. munchies, or any of those sugar/carb highs that'll see us crash. Whenever we have the urge for a snack, we try to step back and ask if we really need it, or if we just mindlessly want it because it's break time and everyone else is having one. Keeping a small bag with ten almonds or a Xocai® chocolate, even a Xocai® protein bar, on hand is one way to be sure of a nice healthy snack whenever one is needed.

A good time to indulge in a healthy snack is before heading out for some event or party. It's all too easy, otherwise, to starve with the notion that there'll be plenty of calories to eat once there. However, whenever we arrive anywhere starved, especially at a buffet table, we're lucky not to sample from every available bowl, plate, and tray. If really hungry, and distracted by a drink or two, we won't even realize what or how much we're eating. So, we eat at least a little something before going. That doesn't mean snack to the point of not eating *anything* once we get there. We just don't arrive so famished as to end up, especially after drinking on an empty stomach, being indiscriminate about our food choices.

Once the time comes when valid WHYs are firmly established in our minds-eyes, good food choices can be better made, no matter where we are. What's more, we suddenly want to make those good choices. There's empowerment in knowing we can control what we put in our mouths, in knowing that we can enjoy, in knowing that we can even recognize that eating that occasional Christmas cookie is okay and not something to fill us with such self-loathing, despair, and/

or sense of failure, that we're inclined to head off for consolatory overindulgence at the nearest feeding trough. We change our life-styles by making better choices, exercising, drinking water, and by letting our taste buds come alive, again, to truly enjoy the good healthy foods that are so much better than the junk food we used to eat.

There's plenty of healthy party food to be had, by the way, even if we make it ourselves and bring it along, asking our hostess first, of course, without making it sound and appear as if we're holier-than-thou.

In our *BACK OF THE BOAT GOURMET COOKING*, we have several recipes that are very healthy party-snack foods....

...like guacamole dip, made by chunking, not mashing, an avocado, along with some diced tomatoes, diced onion, and a dash or more of hot sauce and a splash of lime. By the way, for anyone who has heard that avocados are fattening, their fat has now been determined as "good".

...like fresh salsa with diced tomatoes, onion, jalapeños, a touch of garlic, a splash of lime, a little salt, and a little pepper.

When either of those recipes are combined with some of the healthy organic chips now on the market (first, of course, making sure any ballyhooed fat removal hasn't just been replaced by lots of unhealthy sugar and salt), we're all set. Inexpensive corn chips, from the grocery store, ten chips to a serving, can have surprisingly few calories, especially when teamed with filling fresh veggie dips. By the way, make your own chips from organic tortilla shells or pitas—we especially like the brown-rice ones. Cut those into squares or triangles and bake them. Of course, moderation, as always, is important, even with healthy foods.

Don't forget hummus, or dips made with yogurt or low-fat cottage cheese; all of which can make good and healthy snacking with chips, celery sticks, carrot sticks, and other crudités. We used to make Herbed Goat Cheese Spread, a recipe from our, *BACK OF THE BOAT GOURMET COOKING*, for a crustini, topped with a cucumber round; now, we omit the crustini and put the spread—or hummus—on the cucumber round, instead. We don't miss the crustini, and our bodies don't miss it, either.

Certainly, we try not to use something like a Super Bowl tail-gate party, or *any* party, as an excuse to revert to unhealthy snack habits, especially as there are so many healthy choices from which to choose.

For holidays, for instance, our families, probably like yours, have traditional foods that we prepare. For some reason, it's easy to think that we need to cook enough food, on such occasions, for an entire army. With all that food prepared, we're more apt to pile our plates high. No matter how stuffed we get, we seem to find it necessary to clean our plates so as not to offend our gracious mom, host, or hostess. By making smaller amounts, though, and using smaller dishes, as well as tablespoons instead of serving spoons, we can end up eating much less, no one the wiser.

Certainly, don't fall into the rut of thinking that just because people aren't rolling on the floor, moaning because they're so stuffed, that you didn't do a good job cooking.

For example, Easter at Bruce and Bonnie's house traditionally has been glazed-baked ham, au-gratin potatoes, creamed vegetables, a jellied-type salad (for the kids), and rolls. Strawberry pie and/or shortcake, topped with whipped cream, for dessert. Not wanting to go against tradition, Bonnie, this last Easter, still went for her traditional brown-sugar, blackberry-wine, pineapple-juice, and coca-cola (non-diet) glazed ham. However, where the original recipe calls for one pound of brown sugar, she cut that in half. After the ham was cooked and "resting", she skimmed the fat from the juice in the bottom of the pan before using the defatted juice as a sauce. She eliminated butter from her potato recipe, because there was already enough fat in the cheese to keep the potatoes from boiling to mush in the milk. As for the milk, she could have substituted skim (2% or whole) milk for her recipe's originally called-for cream, but she opted for low-fat unsweetened soy milk, adding more finely diced onions (or chives) to enhance flavor. She eliminated the jellied salad, and, instead, substituted a green salad with finely-diced apples [or orange sections, or grapes], a scant handful of chopped cran-raisins, a tablespoon of finely chopped nuts (to provide the flavor but not the calories of a larger quantity; no longer the candied nuts, once used), it was finished off with a balsamic vinaigrette (heavy on the balsamic, light on the oil). This salad quickly became a child-favorite, because of its fruit and nuts. Likewise, she served a large platter of steamed veggies, spritzed lightly with olive oil, and sprinkled lightly with NapaStyle® Gray Salt, freshly ground pepper, and fresh thyme. No rolls or bread. She eliminated strawberry pie, and, instead, served fresh strawberries, drizzled with "a bit of" balsamic vinegar, "a pinch of" freshly ground pepper, "a bit of" sugar (the berries a little too sour as-was), with "a dollop of" whipped skim milk (flavored with "a pinch of" sugar (or, better yet, Stevia®).

She has taken to the same kind of "cutting down" at her other holiday meals, too, having discovered that mashed potatoes don't need a half a pound of butter, and rich cream, to make them taste good; eliminate the cream, the butter, and ¼ of the calories, but retain the same desired creamy flavor, by substituting sour cream and skim milk. It's not necessary to drown her favorite Green Bean Casserole with cream-of-mushroom soup, either; use fresh mushrooms, wine, and garlic (albeit keeping the French-fried onions—bad Bonnie!).

Any diet-conscious person need only look at his or her traditional holiday fare and see where better choices can be made, by way of ingredients. Still, of course, don't forget to watch portion sizes

That said…don't beat yourself up if and when you do occasionally slip. Merely pick yourself up, dust off, and begin again…as we do.

ENERGY DRINKS, POP, AND CANDY

We warn against "energy drinks", like those commented upon by MSNBC.com, *as "propped up by all sorts of sexy marketing, but not as magical as the ads would have you think. The 'lift' they give you comes from caffeine (nothing fancy there). Some actually have less caffeine than a standard cup of coffee."* One such drink provides 80 mg of caffeine, while a cup of coffee typically delivers 100-150mg. *"The added B vitamins and amino acids are purely for glitz and glam—they don't actually help you perk up. And some varieties are high in sugar, which rushes into your bloodstream and can, ironically, lead to an energy crash in the long run. Not to mention they're an expensive habit to keep up. Bottom line: you're better off drinking a cup of coffee or tea to get your caffeine fix, and if you need a little sweetness, use 1 to 2 packets of sugar or sweetener."* We recommend the natural sweetener Stevia®, easily found at health food stores and, now, at some grocers.

Whatever we do, we stay away from artificially flavored sodas, especially those that are sugar-free; it's still not known what harm some of soda's artificial sweeteners can do us. We just don't want to be guinea pigs. Our bodies aren't artificial, so how can we think they can be benefited by being subjected to each and every artificial ingredient?

We've discovered that Xocai® has a healthy energy drink, Xe®, without added caffeine, or refined sugar, that provides a natural energy boost, without any crash a few hours after drinking it. Occasionally, we drink that.

Often, we bypass energy drinks all together, and opt for a piece, or two, or three of Xocai® the healthy chocolate; no substitutions, please, by any "regular" off-the-counter chocolate ("candy") that's loaded with sugar, fats, fillers, caffeine, even wax; any one of which will likely do us more harm than good. Especially, beware of any candy snack that tries to persuade us that it's healthy just because it contains a high percentage of cacao. In most cases (with the exception of Xocai®, specifically "cold-pressed" to retain nutrients), such advertised-as-healthy cacao is "heat-processed" and has, thereby, lost 70-80% of its natural nutrients; hence, becoming…merely…"candy."

EXERCISE

NOTE: As with dieting, be sure to check with your doctor before starting any kind of exercise program.

There's that often-dreaded word: EXERCISE.

As loathsome as we may find that word, and we often do find it particularly so, it's pretty much necessary in order to reap all of the benefits from any diet program, including this one; we know, because we can't tell you how many times we've tried to lose all of the weight we wanted to lose, without exercise, and never succeeded.

Often, a reason for not exercising is a bona-fide medical one. For instance, after Bonnie was diagnosed as having had her "mini-strokes," she laid around, feeling sorry for herself and getting fat, fatter, fattest, before she realized that she had better get her act together or succumb to death-by-blubber, even if the mini-strokes hadn't killed her. Starting on a diet regime, in order to achieve her objective, was nothing compared to starting exercising.

She started out by walking—on a treadmill—for about a minute and a half a day. Literally, that was all she could manage, at first, and it took her a very long time to work up to twenty minutes. Genuinely, she was proud of herself when she not only managed thirty minutes, but began supplementing those with sit-ups to improve her flabby tummy. That she kept at it was, likely, only because she, admittedly, began feeling so much better, and, of course, delighted in seeing actual results as regarded the reshaping of her body and weight loss.

Then, as bad luck would have it, she took a tumble, chasing her new puppy who had gotten away from her and was about to run into a busy street. Her stumble over one rock saw her lower face hit another. She and Bruce had to spend thousands of dollars putting veneers on her front teeth which, chipped and broken, ripped through her upper lip. The result was several oral surgeries and her inability, for the most part, to have anything but sugar- and fat-laden milkshakes (no Xoçai® shakes available at the time), and eat, more often than not, fattening, soft foods—mashed potatoes, anyone? Her bad diet, plus excruciating headaches, didn't have her feeling much like exercising… or, at least, that became her ongoing mantra.

Only a week after she finally healed from her teeth and mouth injuries, she had yet another medical complication that required additional surgery, putting her back on the couch, again, and back to feeling extremely sorry for herself. Her resumed dormancy saw her gain even more weight. That's where she was, in her life, when she decided it was high time she set to work not only to get back into shape but privately to document that transformation in her personal diary that turned into the fodder for much of this very public book.

Men, as much as women, often have just as many bags of excuses that need to be hauled out with the trash. Bruce stopped exercising at the same time Bonnie did. Like Bonnie, he began to put on the pounds. Like Bonnie, he agreed it was time he got back in shape. They began, drinking Xoçai® shakes which, by then, had become available, and they began eating healthier, including Xoçai® Protein Bars and Xoçai® healthy chocolate.

Although returned to the right pathway by having started up, once again, to make all of the right food choices, and actually losing weight because of it, Bonnie, admittedly, still used her series of surgeries as excuses for not exercising. When she reached a frustrating weight-loss plateau, it was Bruce, who had taken up walking to and from work, who suggested that his wife's failure to lose more weight might well be because she wasn't exercising. He suggested she begin some kind of regular exercise regimen, no matter how low-intensive, to see if that might be the case.

Albeit reluctantly, Bonnie began using the treadmill, pretty much back where she was, months before, when she'd only managed less than a minute-and-a-half whenever she stepped on it, collapsing on the bed for a nap after her minute walk was complete.

Ever so often, while exercising, even today, she still catches herself not breathing, and wonders, "How dumb is that?" However, we've talked to others who say they do the same thing, merely forgetting to breathe while exercising. So, do remember to *breathe correctly.* If we don't, we'll find ourselves gasping for air, as well as getting tired really fast from loss of oxygen, either of which will likely have us ready to throw in our towels before we need to. Bonnie has taken to concentrating on taking deep breaths, and getting air all of the way into her lungs. She can tell she's doing it right when her intakes of air push out her tummy below her belly button—not just push out her chest. To insure correct breathing is taking place, she often puts a hand on her lower stomach, as she breathes in, to verify the very necessary expansion by her lower abdomen. We firmly believe that proper breathing, especially while exercising can provide benefits. Though we may continue to hate exercising, and always needing to be sure we're breathing correctly, we admit, over time, that we have come to enjoy the way exercise makes us look and feel with every drop in weight—and inches.

Admittedly, there are ways we can distract ourselves from the tedious repetition of exercise that has us putting one foot in front of the other. We can watch television. We can listen to music which, when fast-paced, can actually make our feet go faster. Finally, we can play motivational CDs to provide us with whatever additional willpower we may need to keep going.

There's a new exercise, which is actually an old exercise, called "Hooping". Remember the old Hula Hoop? Yup, that's it! Using the hoop is not only fun—and—sometimes very funny—but if you do it for 10 minutes at a time, it's a fabulous exercise that works the whole body. Hooping can be done while watching TV, listening to music, with your family. Kids love it, without even knowing it's good for them! Now, there are even hoops that fold up so we can take them with us.

Finally, Bonnie has reached a point where she actually began enjoying her exercises, if just because of the time it affords her to watch TV, listen to music and CDs; none of which she seemed to manage, even when not laid out on the couch, napping or moping.

We recommend that anyone on a diet start walking, whether on a treadmill, or wherever, until managing at least 10,000 steps a day. Don't guess at that number, either; get a pedometer, like each of us did, and, possibly, be as shocked, as we were, by just how few steps we normally take during the course of any given day. It was a pedometer that convinced Bonnie there was additional walking she needed to do.

Since we had long heard of the wisdom in taking stairs, instead of escalators, or elevators, we started doing just that. We even park our cars at the back of every parking lot, just so we'll have farther to walk to get to a store and back. At first, our legs protested fiercely, but they soon came up to the challenge of providing our minimum 10,000 steps a day.

We can't even begin to tell you how good we began to feel. Not only were we toning our bodies, and adjusting our mental outlook on life, but we were breathing more easily and more correctly than ever.

Doing the same thing, day after day, can sometimes become boring, as well as see us suddenly in "pause" modes, as far as our weight-loss progress is concerned. Adding variety to any exercise regimen can sometimes provide the jump-start needed to get back on track again. We add more distance, walk faster, or jog. Lift weights. Take dancing lessons, which are fun as well as physically beneficial. A thirty-minute workout on the equipment of our local fitness clubs is another good way to go; we drop in on your way home from shopping or after work. Also, we buy exercise DVDs to mix things up bit by following along, with those, instead of exercising by our lonesomes.

Get up and move it, baby.... Move It!

OUR/YOUR JOURNAL

As we've previously mentioned, parts of this book have pretty much been lifted verbatim from Bonnie's personal journal, kept by her as she soul-searched her own WHY for losing weight. By writing down her thoughts, and actions, in black and white, they became more real to her and easier for her to analyze. To this day, each time she finds herself wrestling with her regimen, she reads back through her journal as a way to get herself back into focus.

We recommend everyone keep a journal that includes personal "feelings", regarding dieting ups and downs. Or if you're not the type who wants to put your feelings down on paper, you'll hopefully find reading back through this book, from time to time, whenever you get frustrated, as a way of providing you with the same help it does us by way of getting us back into the grove of self-empowerment and good healthy living.

Definitely, some kind of notebook is needed in which to jot down important statistics of interest, like weight and body measurements. We each prefer a small notebook, with small pen or pencil attached; easy to carry everywhere, so we never have the excuse of not having it readily handy to jot down our food and water intake; and/or steps walked; and/or exercise for the day. We know of others who use PDAs, or cell phones that have places for notes, or smart phones that now have APPs.

Bonnie started out with her beginning weight and waist measurements, and her estimated daily allotment of water. She made the same notations every additional week, in order to see her improvements. Also, as hard as it may sound and seem, she logged in every bite of food and calorie she ate, and we do mean *every* bite and every bit. She was tempted to skip this step, but, without writing everything down that she consumed, the amount was easily forgotten, until fatty thighs quickly jogged her back to the sad reality.

We tend to use any and every excuse for not doing what we're supposed to do, especially regarding our diets; so, we record our food intake (calorie AND portion sizes) as soon after eating as we can. Certainly, we don't wait until we get home, or back to the office, or to a computer, or even to the car. "Food amnesia" is fast-acting; we know. Also, we know that once we got into the habit of keeping track, it got easier to do and provided an invaluable record of how much and how many calories we'd actually eaten—which can be downright mind-blowing and a real eye-opener. Without seeing the actual figures written down on paper, though, we can easily fool ourselves into thinking we're not eating nearly as much as we are.

WEIGHING IN

When we record our weight and waist measurements, each and every week, at the same time of the day, we're sure that we're always wearing the same clothes or no clothes at all. We find it best to do this every Monday morning, immediately after we've gone to the bathroom. If we don't do it then, we're always amazed by how easily we forget, or remember figures as something other (up or down) than they really were. A trick to keep on track over the weekend is knowing that you'll be weighing yourself that coming Monday.

What's more, doing this at the same time, once a week, in the morning, is better for us than doing it each and every day, at various times of the day. Bonnie used to weigh herself many times throughout the day, everyday, as her weight, as everyone's does, fluctuated, according to the time of day, according to the given week, and she wanted to record it when it was on its daily "down", lest she get discouraged. However, once a week, on the same day, at the same time of day, is enough eventually to balance out.

OUR DIET REGIME

The diet we've used for success derives, in part, from recommendations that accompany the official "Xoçai® Protein Shake" diet plan®. Likewise, it includes "eating organic", whenever possible, since we've found that fresh is always best, if not always available. We try to eat whatever fresh fruits and vegetables are in season and whenever, wherever, found, usually at all times of the year, at local farmers' markets. We've found local venders who grow greens hydroponically and organically; unbelievably good. Believe it or not, "frozen" is the next best way to go.

We try to eat only foods that are "natural", not artificial. Meaning, if we are going to eat butter, we eat real butter, only eat less of it than we might normally. Actually, we've come to prefer good-quality organic olive oil, or nutty sesame seed oil. If we're going to use mayonnaise, then we eat real mayo, not "fat-free", only use less of it. We were surprised by how using natural food, that tastes so much better, sees us eating less. We used to put so much fatty mayo on our tuna-fish sandwiches that it actually oozed. Now, we use only about a teaspoon, just enough to moisten the fish, and, believe us when we tell you that we don't miss all of that fatty goop that we've eliminated from our menu.

We try to find local farmers and ranchers by way of acquiring our vegetables, meat, poultry, eggs, and diary products, hormone- and antibiotic-free. We don't need chemicals and toxins as part of our diet. We ask our local grocer specifically about the nature of his products, in that a lot of grocery-men, these days, are wising up to customer demands for more healthy foods. And as more people, like us, and you, buy more healthy foods, the prices for those healthy foods often go down.

When Bruce and Bonnie first started out, they had occasional one-oz. chunks of cheese (even string cheese) by way of high-protein snacks. However, Bonnie proved to be lactose-intolerant. About that same time, they learned from several other people on diets similar to theirs that diary products were the first things to stop eating when reaching a dreaded weight-loss plateau. So, keep cheese in mind, as something possibly to be jettisoned, if a weight-loss plateau suddenly happens to you. Doing so doesn't mean that you'll have to give it up forever, just until you start losing weight again. Of course, as we all come closer to meeting our desired weight-loss goals, no matter what, the rate of dropping ounces automatically, unfortunately, always, seems to slow down.

We started grilling or broiling ground chicken or turkey patties, bagging them, freezing them, and, then, later, popping them in the microwave to provide high-protein snacks. Such 3-oz patties usually contain roughly 160 calories each. We could use regular ground beef, but it has, take note, more fat and more calories.

If we find ourselves at a restaurant that serves huge helpings that we invariably still finish eating, we sometimes ask for half of our meal to be put directly into individual take-home boxes, from the get-go, even before we take our very first bite in the restaurant, leaving us less inclined to open the boxes on-site, more inclined to take them home for later. Of course, nicer restaurants sometimes frown on this, but it's our butts destined to get bigger, not theirs. Then again, nicer restaurants are famous for serving genuinely small portions.

If we don't get at least seven to eight hours of sleep, prescribed as good for optimal health and aiding in weight loss, we end up tired and listless, often thinking, "If we can only eat something, we're sure we'll feel better." Hopefully, we always end up with a piece of fruit, protein, or Xocai® health chocolate.

We did discover, after having not eaten healthy for awhile, then having returned to it, that some gastrointestinal upsets, including diarrhea, bloating, and/or gas can result. These are normal reactions to the reintroduction of fruits and veggies, and their high fiber, into our diets. So we don't use those upsets as excuses to stop. As soon as our bodies start, again, to rid themselves of all the toxic build-ups, and begin to balance out, those conditions go away. In the interim, alleviate some of them by dosing on natural psyllium powder, found in local health-food stores.

WATER

As regards to ounces of water to be drunk by each of us, each day, we each compute our volume on the basis of half our body weight. If, say, Bruce weighs in at 150 pounds, he'll drink at least seventy-five ounces of water a day. Seem a lot? Hey, it's just water, and it's needed to flush the toxins, along with the fat he's losing, out of his system. Peeing is a good thing, even if it is, sometimes, inconvenient. We don't use sudden frequencies of urination as excuses for our not drinking our daily allotments of water. And, in case you're wondering, coffee and tea do NOT count as water. Water is Water is WATER! H_2O.

We've found it easiest to measure out the next day's water on the night before; then, have it all drunk by the end of the next day. There's no need for chug-a-lugging a whole gallon of water at a time, either; we just sip constantly throughout the whole day and stay always properly hydrated. Sometimes, so often on the move, we each divvy up our assigned daily supplies into small glass or stainless-steel bottles, some of which come along with us, wherever we go.

NOTE: Please NO plastic containers. The jury may

still be out on the chemicals presently found in plastics, but why take chances? If some plastics are banned from use in making baby bottles, why should those chemicals be okay for us? Besides, it takes no more time for us to fill glass or metal thermoses, than to fill plastic containers.

CALORIE COUNTS

Presently, Bonnie is on a 1200-1500 calorie-a-day regime; Bruce is on 1500-2000 calories. To some, that might sound like a lot of calories; to others it might sound like not nearly enough. However, when Bonnie eats less, her body seems to go into "starvation mode," always hungry, and she just doesn't lose weight. So, she's discovered, by trial and error, that what her body needs, each and every day, is 1200-1500 healthy non-junk calories.

Not to criticize other diets, but we're of the personal opinions that the problem with a lot of them is that they insist participants, no matter individual metabolisms, eat *less than* 1200/1500 calories. Which can cause weight loss, at first, but, which, eventually, levels off when a dieting body goes into starvation mode; at which point, a dieter is so in need of nourishment that he or she abandons the diet, beats himself or herself up for doing so, only to go back on a diet, yet again, to reach the same starvation-mode plateau as before…on and on…*ad infinitum*. If a few pounds are lost along the way, they're usually soon back.

Bonnie tried one detox diet which required her to

drink some terrible-tasting concoction, supposedly good for her, by way of a ten-to-thirty-day regimen before she even started the diet proper. She ended up "cleansed", all right, but weak and crabby, her body having been flushed clean of nutrients, along with everything else; thereby making her want to eat everything in sight in order to replenish the good stuff lost. She has come to believe that all she really needs to do is replace the junk in her diet with good stuff, and her body takes care of detoxing itself, safely and naturally, without having to endure the torture of any detox-diet's lead-in "flush" regimen.

ORAC

Always, these days, we try to remember that we **DO NOT** need refined sugar. We **DO** need good and healthy fats. We **DO** need good complex carbs, and not from junk-food. We **DO** need high-quality proteins. We **DO** need food with antioxidants; we are firm believers that free radicals **DO** play a major role in weight gain, and in some of the epidemic health issues today, and that antioxidants play a key role in neutralizing those free radicals.

We truly believe that the food most of us eat is so depleted of antioxidants, and nutrition, that we would have to eat all day long to get all we need. That's one reason we prefer Xocai® shakes, protein bars, and/or healthy chocolate, which are the first and, presently, the only high antioxidant meal replacements; soon cookies to be made available. If Xocai® shakes, protein bars, cookies, and healthy chocolate though, aren't your thing, find some other, BUT read labels carefully. If a label doesn't have an ORAC (Oxygen Radical Absorption Capacity) score, which is how to measure antioxidant capabilities to absorb, and/or neutralize free radicals, we don't buy it. We make sure the ORAC score is for the finished product not the ingredients. Some companies tend to fudge on this one, because they know how important antioxidants are, but they don't have the technology to produce a finished product with a high ORAC score. The higher the ORAC score, the better, and, one Xocai® shake is advertised as having as much antioxidants as 100 cups of spinach, or 16 oranges, or 54 cups of carrots, or 40 cups of grapes. We find that incredible. If we originally worried that Xocai® shakes might not provide us with enough fiber, better that we should eat real fruits and vegetables, we discovered Xocai® shakes have all the fiber we need, besides being low-glycemic and lactose-free.

Let us repeat, that we don't advocate eating less real fruits and vegetables, merely that, if you do eat them, you chose those high in antioxidants, like blueberries, artichokes, strawberries, broccoli, broccoli rabe, spinach, and nuts (although, with many nuts, high in fat, do, please, watch those portion sizes).

Even putting an ounce of fresh or organic lemon juice in your water will give you 3200 ORAC.

The more we've learned about antioxidants, and we are certainly beginning to learn more and more, the more we know we're on the right track when including more of them in our menus. Science is even now delving deeper into the healthy properties of cacao beans that were recognized by the Mayans as early as 3000 years ago. Heart, cancer, diabetes, weight gain/loss, high cholesterol, high blood pressure, and, our particular favorite, anti-aging research, and many more health issues, prove, with seeming regularity, the possibly high benefits of some dark chocolate—keeping in mind that not all dark chocolate is created equal.

We each try to consume 100,000 in ORAC per day (The Xoçai® shake has an ORAC value of about 50,000). There's a lot of research about antioxidants and weight-loss, taking up whole books; read some for more extensive detailing on the subject.

We want to be not only thin but healthy, and we want our families that way, too. We have thin friends, and see thin people, who don't "look" healthy, despite their low body weights. Low-fat, or low-carb diets, seem to us, to produce dull hair, dry skin, brain fog, besides all kinds of health issues. Not good! In the mental pictures we always try to have of ourselves, we're not only thin *but* radiantly healthy, with a glow on our cheeks, shiny and healthy hair, and a sparkle in our eyes.

There are major studies being done that seem to confirm the benefits of a high antioxidant diet (GOOGLE "antioxidant") for the prevention—not the cure—of certain health issues (diabetes, high cholesterol, high blood pressure, depression…).

One study, from MD Angerson.org, Jerah Thomas, M.P.H., Peiving Yang, Ph.D., Richard Lee, M.D., and Lorenzo Cohen, Ph.D. says: *"Antioxidants neutralize the electrical charge of free radicals, which damage DNA by taking electrons from other molecules. Free radical damage has been linked to aging and a number of diseases including the development of cancer.*

Antioxidants may slow or possibly protect against cancer.... Research suggests that diets containing antioxidant-rich fruits and vegetables may lower the risk of certain cancers."—http://www2.mdanderson.org/cancerwise/2009/12/what-we-know-about-antioxidants-and-cancer.html

Dark chocolate flavonoids which may play a role in reducing cancer risks are the Cadillacs of the antioxidant world, and occur naturally in the plant-based cacao bean, the base of all chocolate products. Cacao beans are, in fact, one of the most concentrated natural sources of antioxidants. Cacao beans are roasted, ground, and processed to make a variety of different chocolate products. Processing the cacao bean can change the percentage of nutrients left in the final chocolate product.

"Dark chocolate has more of these healthy antioxidants, without the increased sugar and saturated fats that are added to milk," says Sally Scroggs, M.S., R.D., L.D., health education manager in M.D. Anderson's Cancer Prevention Center. *"Now you can eat chocolate without feeling guilty. And that is something everyone can feel good about."*—http://www.mdanderson.org/publications/focused-on-health/issues/2009-february/valentines-sweetest-treat.html

"The amount of antioxidants in your body is directly proportional to how long and healthy you will live."— Dr. Richard Cutler, Anti-Aging Research Development of the National Institute of Health, Washington, D.C.

Most of us love chocolate. By eating healthy chocolate®, like Xoçai®, that isn't laden with sugar, caffeine, waxes, and other "junk," and isn't heat processed to the point of losing its antioxidants and nutrients, we can get our required daily dosages of antioxidants without eating 100 cups of spinach!

SHAKES

We each like a Xocai® Protein Shake every morning, a major meal eaten in mid-afternoon, and, then, especially if we're out to lose weight, another shake, later in the day, protein by way of healthy snacks along the way.

We each start out our day with a Xocai® High Protein Shake, a complete meal, in and of itself, with only 190 calories, that has everything we need for a healthy and complete morning meal. We make it with water and ice, although some people like it with milk [whole, skim, soy, almond, rice, even coconut (which we now hear is good for us)]. Whatever we use in our shake, though, we remember to count the calories.

NOTE: If we do use any liquid other than water for mixing our shakes, we're sure to check the bottle or carton label for sugar content. We were shocked to discover just how much sugar is even in milk, including soy. We look for sugar-free products and buy those whenever possible.

The directions for making a Xocai® High Protein Shake call for 1 cup of water and 2 scoops of powder.

We like to use 1 cup of water and 1 cup of ice. We add a banana, and sometimes even a splash of the syrup usually used to sweeten and flavor lattes. Half a medium banana has about 55 calories, so that makes our shakes with a calorie count of about 245. Sometimes, we add other fruit, even peanut butter, chunky or smooth, for extra protein…or almond butter, an avocado, some coconut, yogurt, coffee, cinnamon, nutmeg, mint, or even Xoçai® Xe® energy drink.

Whatever we add, though, we're sure to count the calories AND WRITE THEM DOWN. We each bought a kitchen scale that allows us to enter a code for whatever food we're going to eat, after which it not only weighs the food but gives us a read-out of its calories, fats, and carbs. This is particularly useful, since not all foods are created equal, by size. Some bananas are long and skinny, some are short and fat. We used to think that if a diet said "one banana" that the banana, of course, needed to be the biggest we could find. Same with oranges, apples, whatever. Of course, that kind of thinking only had us fooling ourselves and sabotaging our diets.

Whenever one of us is intent upon losing weight, faster, he or she often drinks two shakes a day (490 calories), by way of replacing two regular meals; then have Xoçai® chocolates and/or high protein snacks and a meal, making sure to stay within predetermined allotted calorie counts. Some days, a shake can be used as a snack, especially if one of us is going out to a breakfast meeting, and/or to a dinner engagement. This way daily antioxidants and nutrients are kept included, despite what might be served up during the course of the day.

A Xocai® High Protein shake costs less than an average latte, or less than a cup of coffee with doughnut or bagel, and is definitely cheaper than any fast-food breakfast, lunch, or dinner, or prepackaged diet products.

FOOD GROUPS AND RECIPES

We've not provided menus, *per se*. Nor have we stated what foods you should eat with what foods—except to say the fruit is best eaten alone, if it can be. We provide no specific regimen of things to eat, at specific times of each and every day, for a specific number of days, to lose a specific amount of weight. Merely, we provide a selection of food groups and recipes from which to choose, if so inclined, to make-up whatever the daily calorie count *you* judge right for *your* everyday health maintenance and/or weight loss.

You, as well as we, are always perfectly free to substitute healthy foods and recipes not found here, as long as right food choices are recognized, wherever and whenever found, calorie counts always kept, plenty of water drunk, and plenty of exercise accomplished.

Check personal journals or notebooks to see how much is eaten, then pick and choose healthy foods, from the foods available, to round out daily calorie allotments.

We've reduced the calories of our favorite gourmet recipes without compromising taste. Anyone can take a favorite recipe of his or hers and do the same thing simply by using common sense and some healthy tricks.

Whip skim (organic) milk—just careful not to go too heavily on sweetening it, either with sugar, or with Stevia® (a natural sweetener). More than just a pinch or a few drops of the latter, decidedly sweeter than sugar, comes with a thought-by-some-unpleasant "anise" aftertaste.

Add more spices to any dish, and get more taste without more calories.

Use cayenne pepper in food to burn calories—"burn" the operative word here. Cayenne capsules can be bought at local health-food stores.

Use small plates. Smaller portions look larger on smaller plates; it's a trick restaurants learned long ago. Mindlessly, we all tend toward large servings of food on large plates. No need to resort to using saucers, or even luncheon-size plates, though, in that regular dinner plates come in all different sizes—platters, 12", 10", 9"—even smaller. Opt for the smallest size that'll work. Purchase specialty plates and bowls that have really wide rims and small middles; great for smaller portions of soups, and for serving up pastas with sauces, even salads.

Put salad on one side of a plate…a 3-6 oz protein, then a cup or two of veggies, on the other half. It's amazing just how much food that is and how substantial—and satisfying—it looks on a small plate.

Plate directly from the stove or counter, instead

of putting food in serving bowls and platters on the table. This makes it less likely to access convenient seconds…thirds…or….

Use tablespoons, instead of large serving spoons, or ladles, in order to provide smaller servings.

Don't eat at desks, or in cars, not even when rationalizing how eating there will save time; it's a set-up for not paying necessary attention to how much is eaten, and provides an excuse for eating way too quickly. This doesn't mean skip meals altogether, because skipping meals only make us hungrier, with a tendency to overeat the next time we have access to food. Rather, just find the few minutes in every day, in places conducive to relaxation, and eat something then and there. Such times and places are ideal for shakes and protein bars, or a diet cookie, or for other high protein foods which provide sufficient nutrients without taking all that much time out of the day, even when taking the time to chew (thirty-two chews to each bite), and/or to sip slowly a large glass of water. Doing it the right way provides truly good food tastes, as well as a better ability to digest—emphasizing the importance of good planning and having the right kind of snacks on hand, ready to eat.

It's helpful to know the "when" of any celebrations or special events, because forewarned is forearmed, as far as succumbing to the temptations of eating a piece of Auntie's cake, or a slice of Grandma's special pie; better choices having been made by you, for you, before getting there.

RECIPES

SOUPS

Soups fill us up, are easily made, and are usually loaded with good things for us.

Cauliflower Soup

Usually made with cream, you will find this recipe light, yet filling.

1 teaspoon olive oil
1 teaspoon butter
2 leeks, white part only, chopped
1 medium head cauliflower, broken into bite-size florets
1 six-ounce potato, cubed
6 cups chicken stock
Salt and pepper

Melt butter and oil together over medium low heat in a large saucepan.

Add the leeks, cooking until tender, about 10 minutes, stirring frequently. Do not brown.

Turn heat to high.

Add the cauliflower, potatoes, and stock.

Salt and pepper to taste.

Bring to a boil.

Reduce heat, cover, and simmer until vegetables are tender, about 20 minutes.

Remove from heat and cool slightly.

Transfer to a blender and puree.

Transfer to saucepan and bring back to a simmer over medium heat.

If too thick, thin with chicken stock or skim milk (count the calories).

4 servings.

144 calories per servings.

Gazpacho

We love this chilled soup in the summer. It pairs perfectly with the Grilled Tomato Tart and a crisp salad.

6 large Roma tomatoes
1 garlic clove, minced
1 medium cucumber, peeled, seeded and finely diced

½ cup water
1 tablespoon sherry vinegar or red wine vinegar
1 tablespoon olive oil
½ teaspoon Tabasco® sauce
Juice of 1 lemon
Salt to taste
Pinch of cayenne pepper
¼ cup basil, chiffonade or cilantro, roughly chopped

Dip tomatoes in boiling water for 1 minute, remove immediately, and plunge into a bowl of ice water.

Peel, core, remove seeds and chop.

Puree tomatoes, garlic and half of the cucumber in a blender.

Add water, vinegar, oil, Tabasco® sauce and lemon juice, and process until well blended.

Season with salt to taste.

Blend in cayenne pepper.

Cover and refrigerate until chilled, about an hour.

Serve in chilled bowls or large cups.

Garnish with the chopped cucumber and basil or cilantro.

4 servings.

90 calories per serving.

<u>Onion Soup</u>

2 cups leeks, white and pale green parts, chopped, well-washed and drained
1 teaspoon oil olive
¼ pound onion, thinly sliced
¼ pound shallots, thinly sliced
2 cups water
6 ounces potatoes, peeled and diced
1 cup chicken or vegetable stock
2 ounces (½ cup) Gruyère cheese, grated
white truffle oil from www.oilandvinegarusa.com

In the oil, sauté the leeks, onions, and shallots.

Add salt and pepper to taste.

Cook over medium to medium-low heat, until slightly golden brown (about 15 minutes).

Add ½ cup of water to deglaze the pan.

Transfer onions and water to a saucepan.

Add the diced potatoes, stock, and remaining water.

Cover; simmer until potatoes are tender (about 10-15 minutes).

Puree about 1½ cups of resulting soup in a blender,

using caution when blending hot liquids by putting a towel over the blender while it's running.

Stir puree soup back into remaining soup.

Salt and pepper to taste.

Divide into 4 flat bowls.

Sprinkle cheese over soup

Drizzle with truffle oil.

Serve immediately.

Makes 4 servings.

About 170 calories per serving.

NOTE: We like to serve this with Diet Bread Sticks.

Tortilla Soup

1 yellow onion, roughly chopped
1 teaspoon garlic, minced
4 cups chicken or turkey, cut in bite-size strips or shredded
1 twenty-eight-ounce can of tomatoes, organic, petite-cut, diced
6 cups chicken or turkey stock, organic
¼ cup jalapeño peppers, finely diced
2 cups corn, fresh or frozen

- 1 fifteen-ounce black beans, organic, drained, and rinsed
- 2 tablespoons lime juice, fresh
- 2 tablespoons chili powder, organic
- 1 tablespoon ground cumin, organic
- 4 six-inch flour tortillas
- 1 cup Mexican Blend cheese, shredded

Preheat oven to 350°.

In a heavy soup pot, lightly spritzed with oil, and placed on medium-heat, add the onion and garlic.

Sauté until tender but not brown (about 6-7 minutes).

Add the chicken or turkey, tomatoes with juice, the stock, jalapeños, corn, beans, lime juice, cumin, and chili powder.

Bring to a boil.

Reduce heat to low and simmer for about 15 minutes.

Cut the tortillas into thin strips.

Put on baking sheet.

Bake on medium-high until crisp (watch carefully).

Serve in a bowl, topped with tortilla strips and about 1½ tablespoons of cheese.

About 209 calories in a 1-cup serving.

NOTE: We like to serve this with a mixture of baby greens top with ¼ of an avocado, roughly chopped, a squeeze of lime, and salt and pepper to taste.

NOTE: A great way to use leftover turkey or chicken.

SALAD

Pear Salad

2 Bartlett pears, cored and halved
4 cups fresh baby spinach, or arugula or 3 or 4 endive leaves *per serving*
4 teaspoons chopped walnuts or pecans
½ cup Berry Vinaigrette Dressing (See Recipe)
1 oz Bleu Cheese Crumbles

Put the dressing in the bottom of a large bowl and toss with greens.

Thinly slice pears.

Divide into 4 portions.

Top each portion with ¼ of the bleu cheese crumbles and sliced pears. Sprinkle with nuts.

Makes 4 servings.

About 70 calories per serving.

NOTE: If pears aren't in season, and/or are hard, halve

them, and, then, steam for about 3 minutes.

SALAD DRESSINGS

Salads are so good and so good for us. Of course, we're not talking about those awful, chemical-laden, pre-washed, and bagged "things".

It used to be that Bonnie, whenever she went to a nice restaurant, always enjoyed a salad and found it fabulous. While at home, though, her salads always seemed totally blah unless drowned in dressing. It suddenly dawned on her that the difference was that she used packaged salad mixes. Once she started buying her own fresh greens, she never went back again.

A good salad goes way beyond "rabbit food"! Make them with fresh fruits and vegetables that are so good for you, and they will not only keep you thin but healthy.

We particularly love endive and pear salad. At one time, though, Bonnie never bought endive, because she found its by-the-pound price tag seemingly way too expensive. However, experimenting, she realized that she only needed to use 3-5 endive leaves per serving (don't chop or tear), not a whole lot.

By making our own salad dressings, we know exactly what's in them—nothing but good nutrition. Besides which, they are really so easy to make. For most of them, we just put all the ingredients in a jar and shake. Home-made dressing can be stored in the refrigerator in the same jar in which it's made (no metal lids, though, please; this one of the few times plastic, by way of a lid, becomes acceptable, from sheer necessity).

NOTE (and this can't be stressed enough): Put the dressing in the bottom of a serving bowl, and *then* add the greens, etc. Toss the greens with the dressing to coat. This way, we use less dressing than if we drizzle it atop the salad. We can use a spritzer, too, but that only works with dressings like plain vinaigrettes.

Putting a dressing "on the side", for fork-dipping, hardly ever works, in that it's amazing just how much dressing a fork can hold.

Speaking of vinaigrettes, a friend of ours, who owns an Italian restaurant, only serves one salad, delicious, and it's dressed with vinegar and oil. He told us, his dressing is heavy on the vinegar, and light on the oil. What a great idea! Since then, we've been using just enough oil so the dressing sticks to the greens; but not so much vinegar as to overpower the salad. Perfect combination!

Additional experimentation with other dressings provided us with firm evidence that the same culinary trick works just as well with those.

Berry Vinaigrette

1½ cup berries (i.e., raspberries, blueberries, blackber-

ries, boysenberries)
pinch of thyme
¼ teaspoon black pepper, freshly grated
6 tablespoons berry-flavored vinegar (See recipe under "Vinegars")
½ cup water
2 teaspoons oil
pinch of salt
4 drops Stevia®, or 2 teaspoons sugar

Puree all ingredients in a blender until smooth.

Pour into a covered glass jar *(without a metal lid)*.

Cover tightly.

This will keep refrigerated for about 1 week.

Makes about sixteen 2-tablespoon servings.

30 calories per serving.

NOTE: Often, we substitute our berry-flavored vinegar for those flavored and available from www.oilandvinegarusa.com.

Bleu Cheese Dressing

⅔ cup buttermilk
⅓ cup mayonnaise or Yogurt Mayonnaise
½ cup nonfat sour cream
1 tablespoons Worcestershire sauce

1¼ teaspoon dry mustard (Omit if using Yogurt Mayonnaise)
1¼ teaspoon garlic powder
1¼ teaspoon onion powder
1½ tablespoons white vinegar
¼ teaspoon black pepper, freshly ground
½ teaspoon salt
½ cup bleu cheese, crumbled

Combine all ingredients, except bleu cheese, mixing well.

Add cheese and stir gently to combine.

Cover tightly.

Refrigerate for up to 1 week.

65 calories per serving (2 tablespoons)—less if using Yogurt Mayonaise.

<u>Caesar Dressing</u>

Caesar Salads can be super-high in calories. But, by cutting back on the oil, and eliminating the egg yolks, we achieve all of the flavors while eliminating a lot of calories. Also, we choose to eliminate the croutons and really haven't missed them. Then, again, if you think you will miss them, try simply crushing just two or three and sprinkling them on your salad; this provides the flavor while eliminating a good many calories.

1 or 2 anchovy fillets (canned)
1 garlic clove, chopped (more or less, to taste)
½ teaspoon salt
2 egg whites (See Note, below)
¼ cup Parmesan cheese
1 tablespoon lemon juice
black pepper, freshly ground to taste
3 tablespoons extra virgin olive oil
2 medium heads of romaine lettuce

In the bottom of a large, chilled salad bowl, mash the anchovies and garlic with the salt.

Add egg whites, pepper, cheese, lemon juice, and mix well.

Whisk in the olive oil.

Tear the romaine into bit-size pieces. Add to bowl.

Toss gently.

Makes 6 servings

About 90 calories per serving.

NOTE: For safety reason, use pasteurized egg whites, such as Egg Beaters®.

Dijon Yogurt Dressing

½ cup low fat plain yogurt

2 tablespoons skim milk
1 tablespoon Dijon mustard
1 tablespoon scallion, finely minced
Salt and freshly ground black pepper, to taste

Whisk together the yogurt, milk, and mustard.

Stir in scallions and salt and pepper.

Makes 8 servings.

38 calories per 2 tablespoon serving.

Honey-Mustard Dressing

3 tablespoons honey
3 tablespoons Dijon mustard
2 tablespoons extra virgin olive oil
1 tablespoon shallots, minced
1 tablespoon champagne vinegar from www.oilandvinegarusa.com
1½ tablespoons lemon juice (about ½ lemon)
Salt and pepper, to taste

Combine all ingredients until well blended.

Makes 6 servings.

87 calories per 2 tablespoons.

Yogurt Cheese

Empty a carton of plain non-fat yogurt (without gelatin, or other thickeners) into a strainer lined with a double layer of cheesecloth, or paper coffee filter, and place over a bowl.

Cover with wrap and refrigerate overnight.

The consistency of the yogurt cheese will be similar to soft cream cheese. Can be used as a base for dips and spreads, and as a topping for baked potatoes, or anywhere regular mayonnaise, sour cream, or cream cheese is used.

Yogurt Mayonnaise Dressing

¾ cup extra virgin olive oil
1 tablespoon dry mustard
1 teaspoon sugar
1 teaspoon salt
¼ teaspoon Dijon Mustard
3¼ cups yogurt cheese (See instructions for **Yogurt Cheese**)

Gently mix all ingredients in a large bowl until just combined. Don't over mix, or mayonnaise will separate.

Cover tightly.

Will last for about 1 week in refrigerator.

Makes about 1 quart.

55 calories per serving (2 tablespoons).

VINEGAR

Flavored vinegars can add zip to so many recipes. Don't be afraid to use them. We fell in love with balsamic vinegars which vary greatly between brands and age (the older, the milder, and the more expensive).

If you think you don't like vinegars or vinaigrettes, maybe you just haven't tasted the right ones. Experiment with different flavors. We're quite fond of those available from www.oilandvinegarusa.com. You can adjust them to your tastes. Bonnie didn't think she liked vinaigrettes, period, until, too embarrassed to whine that she didn't like them, she condescended to eat one served by her host at a dinner party. To her complete surprise, it was the first time she felt she was "actually eating salad instead of eating dressing." She used to eat a *little* salad with her fat-laden dressing, then wondered why she gained weight after eating *just* a salad.

We've experimented with vinaigrettes and vinegars on a lot of food, by way of garnish. Don't knock it until you try it!

NOTE: In the summer, we've come to love fresh strawberries, blueberries, blackberries and/or raspberries, macerated with a tiny amount of sugar, and a couple splashes of balsamic vinegar and—yes, we really do mean—a grind or two of black pepper. Let it stand for at least twenty minutes (the longer, the better). Fabulous, as a great salad, served on a lettuce leaf or other greens, or, by itself as a light dessert.

Quick Berry Vinegar

1 cup white vinegar
1½ cups berries (i.e. raspberries, blueberries, blackberries, boysenberries)
Pinch of salt

Puree all ingredients in a blender.

Add more vinegar to thin, if needed.

Strain though a sieve.

Store in a glass jar or bottle *(without metal top or lid)*.

Refrigerate.

NOTE: If you don't mind the berry seeds, don't strain. We often don't strain our blueberries, because we enjoy the bits of berries and seeds add to the dressing.

NOTE: This can be made with other fruits too, such at pineapple, mangoes, lemons, oranges, etc.

VEGETABLES

Believe it or not, a lot of vegetables are "free" foods, in that our bodies burn more calories digesting them than the number of calories they provide. Therefore, we can eat as much of these as we want. Yes, even five cups of broccoli, if that sounds good to you. Personally, we like broccoli, but five cups as one serving just might be overdoing it. However, if you don't like any veggies, *get over it*. Learn to like them.

You're a new person now, naturally thin and healthy; so, eat like one. Remember, it's the foods you *were* eating, and liking, that made you an unhealthy, fat, and miserable person. Learn to like good, wholesome foods, like some of these vegetables:

Asparagus
Artichokes
Broccoli
Brussels spouts
Cabbage
Celery
Cucumbers
Eggplant
Fava Beans

Green beans
Green, red, yellow peppers
Jícama
Lettuce/greens
Mushrooms
Radishes
Spinach
Sugar pea pods
Tomatoes

   The vendors at farmers' markets often let us sample their veggies and fruits. That's always a great way for us to find new ideas and new tastes. We are careful, like with everything else, to check the calories. If we are indulging in fresh veggies, we're sure they're not the starchy, high calorie ones.

   Frozen vegetables are best when fresh isn't available, in that frozen vegetables are picked ripe and frozen soon afterwards, so they retain a lot of there goodness.

   Surprisingly, most "fresh" produce in grocery stores isn't fresh at all, having been shipped miles to the stores; so it's usually harvested before it's ready—in—some cases, totally green. Then, it's often sprayed with some kind of ripening agent so it ripens en route. If you've experienced produce seemingly rotting overnight, blame the ripening agent still at work!

   One solution we've found, when forced into buying non-local produce, is to give it a quick rinse, then a quick dunk in a solution of water mixed with 1 tablespoon (more or less depending on the size of your container) of bleach; then, another quick rinse, and a drain. We find our produce lasts a little longer, if we do this. Also, there are produce washes available on the market.

NOTE: Strawberries should never be washed until you're ready to eat them, as they don't keep after washing. We never bleach-rinse them, either. Buy them fresh, wash them, and eat them immediately.

Veggies are best eaten raw, steamed, or grilled, never boiled which depletes them of nutrients. For grilling, use a drizzle or a spritz of olive oil, then toss to coat. You can get an oil spritzer at any kitchen supply store. Don't use those aerosol cooking sprays, as they're mostly chemicals. Use good organic oils, preferably olive oil; extra virgin, for salads, breads, veggies, etc; regular olive oil for cooking.

We love to grill most anything, even garlic or scallions. By way of finish, just sprinkle on your favorite fresh herbs.

A particular favorite is sugar-pea pods, or fava beans in their pods, spritzed with oil, grilled in a grill pan, over medium heat, so they "steam" until the outside is slightly brown. Great for a snack or side dish, after removing the fava beans from their pods; the sugar-pea pods are edible.

Artichokes and green, yellow, and red peppers, need to be prepared, first, before grilling. See *BACK OF THE BOAT GOURMET COOKING* for the how-to, careful not to overcook and lose the nutrients.

Even some frozen veggies can be grilled.

Green Bean Casserole—Bonnie Style
(Adapted from NapaStyle®/Michael Chiarello)

Onion Straws (See recipe below)
1 pound green beans
1 tablespoon olive oil
½ lb mushrooms, roughly chopped into bite-size pieces
2 garlic cloves, finely minced
2 teaspoons thyme, finely minced
Salt and pepper to taste
⅓ cup red wine
⅓ cup chicken or vegetable broth

Put beans in a streamer basket over simmering water for about 7 minutes or until tender.

Remove from water and set aside.

In a sauté pan, heat oil over medium heat.

Add mushrooms. Do not stir or turn until they start to caramelize, then turn and cook until nicely caramelized. If you stir them too soon, they release their juices then just boil.

Add the garlic, thyme, salt and pepper.

Cook until garlic starts to brown. Do not overcook.

Reduce heat, add the wine and broth, and cook for about 2-3 minutes.

Add the green beans and toss lightly.

We like to serve these on a platter with a raised sides.

Top the Onion Straws.

Onion Straws

1 large onion
4 cups vegetable oil for deep frying
½ cup buttermilk (See Note)
1 cup flour

Thinly slice onion, using a mandoline, as if slicing for French Onion soup.

Cut the onion rounds in half and separate.

Put in a bowl (with a tight lid).

Pour buttermilk over onions and soak for about 30-60 minutes, turning over often.

Heat oil to 350°F.

Drain onions and dip into the flour, and *immediately* drop into the oil.

Fry about 1 minute (until crispy), watching closely; these are thin and will burn quickly.

Drain on a paper towel.

Set aside in a warm place (a warming oven if possible). Do *not* keep warm in a low oven; they'll get soggy.

Makes 4 large servings.

Calorie count (approx 100 per serving) varies because of possible degrees of flour on the onions that affects the oil absorption.

NOTE: We always have powdered butter milk on hand, following the directions on the package to make ½ cup.

Grilled Tomato Tarts

Tart Shells

1 cup flour
¼ teaspoon salt
1 large egg
2 tablespoons olive oil
1 tablespoon water

In a food processor, pulse together the flour and salt.

With the motor running, add the egg, oil, and water.

Pulse until just combined but still crumbly.

Remove from processor and gently pat in to flatten ball.

Cover with plastic wrap and chill for 30 minutes, or until well chilled.

Topping

3 large ripe tomatoes, peel removed, sliced paper thin
2 tablespoons fresh grated Parmesan cheese
Salt, preferably NapaStyle® Gray Salt
Freshly ground pepper
2 tablespoons fresh basil leaves, chiffonade or cilantro, roughly chopped

Preheat grill to medium heat.

Roll pastry dough to about ⅛" thick on a lightly floured surface.

Cut four 6" circles and prick with a fork.

Turn grill to low.

Turn off flame directly under pastry.

Lightly oil the grill grates.

Carefully place on grill for about 5 minutes until crisp, but not brown. Watch closely as they burn easily.

Remove from grill, place grilled side up.

Put tomato slices overlapping, completely covering the pastry, about ½" from edge.

Sprinkle with the cheese, salt and pepper to taste.

Return to grill.

With grill lid down, grill until tomatoes are cooked and pastry is slightly brown, about 5 more minutes, watching closely to make sure they don't burn.

Remove from grill.

Sprinkle basil or cilantro on top.

Makes 4 servings

195 calories per tart.

A wonderful accompaniment to Gazpacho.

NOTE: With only small variations, these can also be made in the oven:

Preheat over to 375°.

Bake pastry rounds for about 5 minutes.

Remove from oven.

Add sliced tomatoes, cheese, salt, and pepper.

Bake for about 5-8 minutes until tomatoes are cooked.

Remove from oven.

Sprinkle with basil and cilantro.

Potatoes

Potatoes are usually a big no-no on most restricted diets. Potatoes, though, are loaded with vitamins and nutrients, and, if prepared without frying or deep frying, and without being loaded with heaps of butter, sour cream, cheese, bacon, or dunked in globs of tarter sauce, can, in moderation, be eaten, on occasion. In fact, a baked potato makes a wonderful lunch, or a light dinner, with a salad with vinaigrette.

Top with:

About a cup of salsa, a tablespoon of grated Monterey Jack or Cheddar cheese, and a little onion

Or…

2 tablespoons of sour cream, a tablespoon of crisp, crumbled bacon, sprinkling of chives,

Or…

A cup of roughly chopped broccoli, with a tablespoon or 2 of grated cheese, put under the boiler for a minute to melt the cheese,

Or…

¼ cup of chili, a tablespoon or two of grated cheese

and a sprinkling of chopped onions

All of the above have about 190 calories for a small potato, about 325 calories for a medium potato, or about 515 for a large potato.

Oven-Roasted Garlic and Herb Potatoes

2 lbs baby red or Yukon Gold potatoes
olive oil in a spritzer
4 garlic cloves, finely minced
1 teaspoon each rosemary, thyme, and oregano
NapaStyle® Gray Salt
Black pepper, freshly ground

Preheat oven to 450°.

Scrub potatoes.

Leave skins on and cut into large chunks.

Put on a lightly oiled baking sheet—with sides.

Spritz with oil, but don't overdo.

Sprinkle with the minced garlic and herbs.

Toss to coat thoroughly.

Bake for 15 minutes; then, turn and bake 15 minutes more, until browned and crisp.

Salt and pepper to taste.

Makes 4 servings of ½-pound each.

About 197 calories per serving.

Spinach Soufflés

These are low in fat. Made in 8-oz ramekins, they're a great lunch, served with a salad and the Diet Bread Stick. Made in 4-oz ramekins, they make a good side dish.

½ cup bread crumbs, freshly made and dried in moderately heated oven about 2 minutes
½ teaspoon butter, melted
5 oz fresh spinach
Salt and freshly ground pepper, to taste
1½ tablespoons cornstarch
1⅓ cup skim milk
¼ cup Gruyère cheese, grated
3 large egg whites
Pinch of cayenne pepper
Pinch of fresh grated nutmeg

Preheat oven to 400°.

Lightly oil 4, four-oz ramekins.

Sprinkle with bread crumbs, coating bottom and sides, shaking out any excess.

Place ramekins on a baking sheet.

Wash thoroughly and removed stems of spinach.

Shake off water and add spinach to a lightly buttered, non-stick sauté pan.

Salt and pepper.

Cover and cook over medium heat for about 2 minutes, or until spinach has wilted.

Remove from heat and drain in a fine sieve, pressing out excess liquid.

Puree spinach in a blender.

Transfer to a bowl.

In a small saucepan, gradually whisk milk into cornstarch until smooth.

Place over medium heat and bring to a boil, whisking frequently.

Reduce heat to medium low, cook, whisking frequently, until very thick, about 3 minutes.

Remove from heat. Whisk in Gruyère cheese, nutmeg, and cayenne.

Add to spinach and mix well.

Beat the egg whites on medium speed until firm peaks form.

Beat in about ¼ of the spinach mixture, blending well.

Using a rubber spatula, carefully fold in the remaining spinach mixture.

Divide between the prepared ramekins, filling about 3/4 full.

Reduce oven to 375°.

Bake for 20 minutes, or until center is firm when you tap lightly on the ramekin, and the top is lightly golden.

Serve immediately.

Makes 8 4-oz or 4 8-oz soufflés.

74 calories per 4-oz soufflé (148 calories per 8-oz soufflé).

Steamed Vegetable Platter

One of our favorite lunches, or even a light dinner, is a large plate of steamed vegetables—broccoli, cauliflower, carrots, green beans, asparagus, zucchini, or whatever your favorites.

The different vegetables cook at different times. It also depends on the thickness of the vegetables, but most will cook in 5 to 15 minutes.

You will need a large pot and a steamer basket that will fit inside.

Fill the pot with enough water so that it is just barely below the bottom of steamer basket.

Once the water comes to a boil, put the carrots and cauliflower in first, and steam for about 3 minutes before adding the other vegetables that take a little longer to cook.

Cover with lid.

Steam until *al dente* (about another 3 to 5 minutes).

Drain, reserving about 2 tablespoons of the cooking liquid.

Put vegetables on a warm platter (You can warm platter by rinsing with hot water).

Melt ½ teaspoon of butter in the reserved water and pour over vegetables.

Salt and pepper to taste, using fresh ground pepper and NapaStyle® Gray Salt.

Serve immediately.

FISH AND SEAFOOD

Fish is one of the best "diet" foods there is. Low in calories. High in protein. Low in fats. Some are loaded with healthy Omegas, essential oils, vitamins etc.

Just, please, don't ruin good fish by breading and, then, deep-frying it.

And, please, forget the tarter sauce No need if you use fresh-squeezed lemon or **Lemon Sauce** (See our recipe).

You can place the fish on a bed of steamed fresh spinach, or kale, with or without (frozen) lima or fava beans by:

Simply sautéing 1 thinly sliced garlic clove in a teaspoon of olive oil, until fragrant, but not brown.

Add freshly washed greens, don't shake off water. The water on, and in, the greens will provide for the "steaming".

If using the frozen beans, add a package of them and about 1 tablespoon of water.

Cover and cook until greens are just wilted.

Transfer to plates, top with fish.

Serve immediately with freshly squeezed lemon or our **Lemon Sauce**.

NOTE: Steamed greens are, also, good with chicken.

Finally, DO realize that fish doesn't naturally come "with fries."

Mostly, we prefer our fish *au naturel*, with just a little salt (preferably NapaStyle® Gray Salt), ground pepper (or lemon pepper, or our **Spice Rub**—for the latter, See our Recipe), instead of breading.

NOTE: Our **Spice Rub** works well with fish, chicken, grilled vegetables, pork…or use a pinch or two in soups or scrambled eggs.

Spice Rub

1 cup of fennel seeds
2 tablespoons coriander seeds
2 tablespoons black peppercorns
3 tablespoons coarse salt, preferably NapaStyle® Gray Salt
2 tablespoons paprika
1 teaspoon cayenne

Over medium heat, put the fennel seeds, coriander seeds, and peppercorns in a small heavy skillet.

Toss the seeds frequently, toasting evenly.

Watch carefully, so as not to burn.

Cool on a plate before grinding (warm seeds will gum up the grinder).

When seeds are cool, in small batches, grind with the salt until all the seeds are finely ground.

Pour into a bowl, with the paprika and cayenne; mix well.

Store in an airtight container in a dark and cool place for about 3 months, or in freezer for about a year.

NOTE: We use a coffee grinder that we keep just to grind spices in small batches.

Crab Quesadilla with Avocado

Pico de Gallo

4 Roma tomatoes
2 jalapeño peppers, seeds and veins removed, finely diced
1 small red onion, finely diced
2 tablespoons lime juice
½ teaspoon garlic, finely minced
¼ cup cilantro leaves, roughly chopped and loosely pack
½ to ¾ teaspoon salt, preferably NapaStyle® Gray Salt

Pepper, freshly ground to taste

Mix lightly together and set aside.

NOTE: If you like it hotter, leave the seeds and veins in the jalapeños.

Quesadilla

4 nine-inch flour tortillas
4 teaspoons diced canned green chili peppers
½ cup chopped crab meat
½ cup low-fat Monterey Jack cheese, grated
½ cup diced avocado
Salt and pepper to taste
¼ cup sour cream

Top ½ of each tortillas with 4 tablespoons Pico de Gallo.

Divide the avocado, green chilies, crab, and cheese on each tortilla.

Salt and pepper to taste.

Fold in half.

Lightly spritz a large sauté pan with oil.

Heat over medium heat.

Cook each tortilla 3-5 minutes on each side (until

cheese is melted).

Cut into 3 triangle pieces.

Serve with 2 tablespoons Pico de Gallo and 1 tablespoon of sour cream on the side.

Makes 4 servings.

395 calories per serving.

Poached Salmon with Orange Relish

Orange Relish

1 cup orange segments, roughly chopped, with juice
3 tablespoons fresh basil chiffonade (finely cut strips)
½ cup red onion, finely diced
1½ tablespoons jalapeño pepper, seeds and veins removed, finely diced
1½ teaspoons olive oil
¼ cup red wine vinegar
1 teaspoon salt
½ teaspoon freshly ground black pepper

Mix all ingredients together and set aside.

Poached Salmon

1½ cup fresh orange juice
½ cup water
1 tablespoon grated orange peel

1 cup white wine (or chicken stock)
4 four-ounce salmon fillets

Over high heat, combine orange juice, water, orange peel, and white wine (or chicken stock) in a pan large enough to hold the salmon, without overcrowding.

Bring to a boil.

Reduce heat to medium low and *carefully* add fillets, one at a time, using a slotted spoon.

Bring liquid back to a simmer, *do not boil*.

Cover and remove pan from heat.

Let stand for 10 minutes.

Check for doneness.

Remove with a slotted spoon.

Serve with Orange Relish

Make 4 servings

270 calories per serving

Salmon with Berry Vinaigrette

4 four-ounce salmon fillets
½ cup **Berry Vinaigrette** (See our recipe).

Salt and freshly ground pepper, to taste.

Heat a cast-iron pan, big enough for all 4 fillets, on a grill preheated to medium-high.

Brush fillets with vinaigrette on both sides, using 2 tablespoon on each fillet.

Marinate for about 15 minutes. *Do not marinate any longer* or the vinegar in the marinade will start to cook the salmon and make it mushy.

Remove pan from grill, lightly oil, put back on grill.

Add fillets.

Cook about 3-4 minutes (until cooked about half way though).

Turn and cover lightly with a piece of foil.

Close lid on grill.

Cook 5 more minutes (until cooked through; careful not to overcook).

Remove to a warm platter.

Add any leftover marinate with a splash of lemon juice to the pan.

Heat thoroughly, and pour over fillets.

Serve immediately.

Makes 4 servings.

237 calories per serving.

NOTE: Can be prepared on top of stove and finished in a 350° oven.

<u>Sole with White Wine and Grapes</u>

1 tablespoon olive oil
1 pound sole fillets, no skin and boned
½ cup flour
Salt and freshly ground pepper, to taste
1 teaspoon butter
½ teaspoon rosemary, finely chopped
1 cup dry white wine (or chicken stock)
½ cup red grapes, seedless and cut in half

Heat oil over medium high heat.

Season fillets with salt and pepper and dredge in the flour, removing any excess.

Cook in oil for about 4 minutes on one side, turn and cook for minute.

Transfer to a platter or plates.

Keep warm.

Turn heat to medium.

Slightly brown butter.

Add rosemary.

Stir for about 30 seconds.

Add wine (or chicken stock) and deglaze the pan, scraping the bottom of the pan.

Turn heat to medium low and reduce wine to half.

Add grapes to warm.

Spoon sauce over fish.

Serve immediately.

Sole Stuffed with Crab

4 four-ounce sole fillets

Stuffing

1 cup jumbo lump crab meat
1 tablespoon mayonnaise
¼ cup red bell pepper, finely diced
1 tablespoon Italian parsley, freshly chopped
Salt and freshly ground black pepper, to taste

Bread-Crumb Topping

1 garlic clove, finely minced
2 teaspoons oil olive
¼ cup fresh bread crumbs, fine
1 teaspoon lemon zest, finely grated

Preheat oven 450°.

Mix crab, mayonnaise, red bell pepper, parsley, salt, and pepper.

Lay sole flat, dark side up.

Season with salt and pepper.

Divide the crab mixture, mounding on the fat end of the fillet.

Fold the other end over the stuffing, tucking the end underneath to form a bundle.

Set aside.

In a 9" oven-proof sauté pan, with a lid, heat the minced garlic and oil over medium heat for about 30 seconds.

Add the bread crumbs, then cook and stir until golden brown.

Remove from heat; stir in lemon zest.

Lightly salt and pepper.

Transfer to a dish.

Put the fillets in the pan, and sprinkle with the breadcrumb mixture.

Bake in the upper part of the oven for about 20 minutes.

Uncover and put under broiler for a minute or two to crisp bread crumbs.

Carefully transfer fillets to plates, reserving the juices.

Deglaze

Place pan over medium high heat.

Add ½ teaspoon of butter and 1 tablespoon lemon juice.

Stir vigorously to dislodge pan-stuck bits.

Drizzle over fillets.

Makes 4 servings.

About 210 calories a serving

DAIRY

Marinated Goat Cheese

Goat cheese has a zesty flavor. If you have not tried it, do. Marinated and served on the side of the plate with a mixed green salad with a vinaigrette dressing and a couple of Diet Bread Sticks, it makes a perfect lunch or a lovely summer's dinner.

This recipe makes a perfect low-calorie appetizer, or snack spread, on a cucumber slice (round), or in the hollow of a stalk of celery. It, too, can make a lovely salad layered between juicy ripe tomato slices resting on a bed of crisp lettuce, or romaine leaf.

NOTE: This recipe can easily be halved.

5-oz log fresh goat cheese
3 garlic cloves, minced
2 tablespoons extra virgin oil olive
1 teaspoon fresh thyme leaves
Black pepper, freshly coarse-ground

Slice goat cheese log into ten ½ ounce disks.

Put in a shallow glass dish in a single layer.

Combine the minced garlic with the olive oil and thyme.

Drizzle over the cheese rounds.

Generously season with the freshly coarse-ground black pepper.

Cover and refrigerate for at least 2 hours.

Will last in the refrigerator for up to 2 days.

Makes 10 servings.

67 calories per serving.

FOWL

Just because we eat a lot of chicken doesn't mean we have to eat dry, leather-like chicken. While we prefer chicken breasts, boneless thighs can be used.

If you tend to avoid chicken breast because of their dryness, you'll be surprised how cooking them properly—not overcooking—will win you over.

We usually take half of a chicken breast, cut in half, lengthwise, butterflied, and put between two sheets of plastic wrap.

Pound until thin. (Depending how we plan to cook the chicken, we'll either remove the skin, or leave it on).

Sear or grill in pan.

Salt and pepper to taste.

With a wedge of lemon, serve on a bed of steamed spinach, or on, or with a salad.

Or....

Preheat oven 350°.

Lay chicken breasts out flat.

Pile on a few fresh spinach, chard, or kale leaves.

Add a tablespoon of grated cheese of your choice, we prefer Parmesan.

Salt and pepper.

Roll up and secure with toothpicks.

Put in an oven-proof pan.

Bake for about 20 minutes, until juices run clear, being careful to not overcook.

Transfer to a platter or plates.

Keep warm.

Over high heat, deglaze pan with a splash or two of dry white wine.

Pour over chicken.

Serve immediately.

Or....

Roll up 3 or 4 *frozen* asparagus spears in the flattened

chicken breasts (Do not use *fresh* asparagus spears, in that they'll cook much faster than the chicken and will overcook and turn black).

Salt, preferably NapaStyle® Gray Salt, and pepper.

Bake in a preheated 350° oven for about 30 minutes.

Transfer to a platter or plates.

We used to serve a hollandaise sauce with this, but now we simply….

Brown 1 teaspoon butter in the same pan in which the chicken was cooked.

Deglaze the pan with white wine.

Drizzle over chicken.

Serve immediately.

Or….

Serve with our **Lemon Sauce**

Or….

Heat about a tablespoon of oil in a large skillet.

Sprinkle each flattened breast with a pinch or two of our **Spice Rub**.

Quickly brown on each side for about 2-3 minutes over medium high heat (Do not overcook).

Transfer to a platter or plates.

Add a pinch or two of rosemary or thyme to the pan.

For each piece of chicken use about ½ cup of red wine and ½ cup chicken stock to deglaze the pan (or 1 cup stock).

Reduce liquid to about ½.

Add 5 red grapes cut in half for each piece of chicken.

Heat through.

Pour over chicken.

Serve immediately.

Or....

Same as above, only substitute white wine and green grapes.

Honey-Pecan Crusted Chicken

2 chicken breasts, medium-size, boneless
2 tablespoons Dijon mustard
Pinch each of thyme, cumin, paprika, and cayenne
1 tablespoon honey, optional

1 egg white
1 tablespoon fresh lemon juice
1 cup Panko crumbs
¼ cup pecans, finely chopped
Pinch of garlic powder or fresh minced garlic
½ teaspoon salt
Freshly ground black pepper, to taste

Preheat oven to 350°.

Slice each breast in half lengthwise down the center.

Dampen slightly with water.

Cover with a piece of plastic wrap.

Lightly pound each piece to make even thickness.

Whisk together, in a pie plate, the mustard, herbs, honey, egg white, and lemon juice; set aside.

In a separate pie plate, mix well, the bread crumbs, pecans, garlic or garlic powder, salt and pepper.

Dip the chicken in the mustard mixture.

Roll mustard-dipped chicken into crumb mixture, pressing crumbs on both sides.

Let the breaded chicken air-dry on a rack for a few minutes to prevent crumbs from falling off while sautéing.

Lightly spritz an oven-proof nonstick pan. (We use a well-seasoned cast-iron pan)

Heat oiled pan on medium heat, and sauté chicken about 3 minutes (until golden brown).

Carefully turn chicken, put pan in preheated oven, and roast until cooked through, about 8-10 minutes.

Transfer to a platter or plates.

Scrape the crumbs from the bottom of the pan and sprinkle over the chicken.

Makes 4 servings.

About 260 calories per serving.

Slice and serve on top of mixed greens dressed with our **Honey-Mustard Dressing** (an additional 231 calories for a total of 490 calories).

In the winter, we omit the honey and serve over a bed of steamed spinach, chard, or kale, with a drizzle of lemon; streamed veggies on the side.

Inside-Out Turkey Burgers

1 lb ground turkey
¼ cup Gruyère cheese, finely grated
4 scallions, finely minced
¼ cup Dijon mustard

1 garlic clove, minced
Salt and freshly ground pepper

Heat grill to high.

In a bowl, combine the turkey, cheese, scallions, mustard, garlic, salt and pepper, careful not to over mix (makes burgers tough).

Form above mixture into 4 patties.

Sear patties quickly on both sides (about 1 to 2 minutes per side).

Turn heat to medium (or move patties to a cooler part of the grill).

Cook 5-7 minutes per side (until done; do *not* overcook).

Makes 4 servings.

253 calories per serving without a bun; otherwise, calories with bun depend upon what type of bun is used—so, add calories accordingly.

Tetrazzini (Chicken or Turkey)

This is a great way to use leftover turkey or a deli-roasted chicken.

2 tablespoons butter

½ lb mushrooms, sliced
⅓ cup flour
1¾ cup chicken stock
1⅓ cup skim milk
½ teaspoon NapaStyle® Gray Salt
¼ teaspoon black pepper, coarsely ground
⅛ teaspoon fresh nutmeg, grated
3 cups (1 lb) chicken, skinless, boneless, shredded
½ lb spaghetti
½ cup Parmesan cheese, grated

Preheat oven to 425°.

Lightly oil a 9"x13" baking dish.

Cook spaghetti according to directions on package—al dente.

In a large nonstick skillet, melt butter over medium high heat.

Add mushrooms to pan, but do not stir until they start to brown, about 2 minutes; stir and sauté for another 2 minutes until brown.

Stir in flour with the mushrooms.

Add the broth and milk.

Cook, stirring until mixture comes to a boil.

Reduce heat.

Stir constantly until mixture thickens (about 2 minutes).

Add nutmeg, salt and pepper to taste.

Remove from heat.

Add chicken and spaghetti.

Toss lightly.

Spoon into the prepared baking dish.

Sprinkle with the Parmesan cheese.

Bake 20 minutes (until golden brown and bubbly).

Serves 8.

281 calories per serving.

SAUCES

Lemon Sauce

This sauce is good served with most any kind fish. We especially like it with salmon.

Put a puddle of about 2 tablespoons of it on a plate and lay the fish on it. Also, it works great when drizzled over some vegetables, especially asparagus and puddled under or drizzled over chicken.

1 teaspoon butter
1 tablespoon flour
½ cup chicken stock
¼ cup skim milk
1 teaspoon lemon zest
2 tablespoons lemon juice, fresh
NapaStyle® Gray Salt and freshly ground pepper

In a small sauce pan, melt and slightly brown the butter over medium heat.

Whisk in the flour.

Cook about 2 minutes.

Reduce the heat.

Slowly whisk in the chicken stock and milk.

Simmer until thickened, whisking constantly.

Add the lemon juice.

Salt and pepper to taste.

Cook about 2 minutes more.

Makes about 1 cup.

10 calories per tablespoon.

Turkey (or Chicken) Gravy

1 teaspoon butter
½ cup chopped onion
1 celery stalk, minced
2 tablespoons flour
1 cup turkey or chicken stock
½ cup evaporated skim milk
½ cup water
Salt and freshly ground black pepper, to taste

Heat the butter over medium high heat.

Lower heat to medium low.

Add onion and celery.

Cook until tender, stirring occasionally.

Sprinkle flour in the pan, over the vegetables.

Stir until the flour is brown (about 3 or 4 minutes).

Whisk in broth, milk, and water.

Bring to a boil.

Lower heat and simmer until thickened (about 10 minutes).

Strain to remove the vegetable, or puree in blender. (Depending on what we are serving this with, we may not remove or puree the vegetables).

Salt and pepper to taste.

This freezes well.

Makes 8 servings.

34 calories per serving.

NOTE: Substitute vegetable or beef broth for the turkey, or chicken broth, or omit milk and use 1½ cups broth. If you have roasted a turkey—or chicken—skim off the fat. You can also omit the veggies as the drippings already have lots of flavor.

NOTE: Because it is low calorie doesn't mean you

have to "pour" it on. Just drizzle a tablespoon or two over the food, or puddle on the plate under the food; after all, it is only supposed to complement the food, not be a meal unto itself.

PASTAS

Yes, it is possible to eat pasta on a diet! *Just* watch your portions.

We try to stay away from cream sauces, but if a recipe calls for heavy cream, we use low fat or even skim. As Bonnie doesn't eat "much" dairy, we substitute sugar-free soy, or rice milk. She didn't notice any difference, and her Mother who, being a fabulous, but old-school cook, who would never consciously let soy touch her lips, didn't know the difference, either.

Rest assured that if Bonnie's Mother didn't know, we doubt anyone one else will either! Not that we were trying to put over anything on her, but if we even mention using soy milk instead of cow's milk, she always brings cow's milk with her.

Calories vary as to the kinds of pasta we're cooking—fresh versus dry, egg noodles, spaghetti, spiral, etc. Read the label. Rule of thumb is 2 ounces of uncooked, dry pasta equals about a cup cooked. One cup of cooked pasta is a serving size.

Make your sauces with fresh ingredients, making for a quick and easy sauce. If using canned ingredients, make sure they're organic.

<u>Lemony Herb Pasta</u>
(Adapted from our
BACK OF THE BOAT GOURMET COOKING)

Prepare ½ pound spaghetti according to directions on the package. (2 ounces equals a 1 cup serving.)

Drain, reserving pasta water.

Lemon-Herb Sauce

1 tablespoon olive oil
3 cloves of garlic, finely minced
½ cup Italian parsley, roughly chopped
1 teaspoon thyme leaves, fresh
Juice of ½ lemon
1 teaspoon lemon zest
Parmigiano Reggiano or Parmesan cheese

Heat olive oil over medium heat.

Turn heat to low, and add minced garlic.

Sauté until slightly brown, watching carefully.

Add the cooked pasta and enough pasta water to make a sauce.

Add the lemon juice, parsley, thyme, and lemon zest.

Toss lightly.

Sprinkle with grated cheese.

Makes about 4 servings.

256 calories per serving.

NOTE: If our daily calories allotments allow it, we sometimes add 3 or 4 cooked shrimp, or 3 ounces grilled chicken. Shrimp and chicken can be grilled kabob-style and served atop the pasta. Just be sure to count those calories.

Sun-Dried Tomato and Sausage Pasta

8 ounces whole wheat rigatoni or spaghetti
2 Italian sausage, hot or sweet, cut into about 10 pieces each
1 tablespoon olive oil
1 medium yellow onion, rough chopped
2 cloves garlic, minced
1 fourteen-ounce can tomatoes, petite diced, organic
2 halves, jarred, sun-dried tomato, julienne
1 to 2 tablespoons Italian seasoning, to taste
Salt and pepper to taste

Cook pasta according to directions on package—al dente, reserving some of the pasta water.

In a pan, heat oil over medium heat.

Add sausage and onions, until brown.

Add garlic and cook about 1 minute.

Add sun-dried tomatoes, stirring quickly to release oil.

Stir in tomatoes with juice, Italian seasoning, salt and pepper.

Turn heat to low and simmer while pasta cooks, about 10-12 minutes.

Add cooked pasta to sauce, using reserved pasta water, if needed, to make the sauce thinner; add squirts of tomato paste to make it thicker.

Serve immediately.

Makes 4 servings.

About 382 calories per serving.

BREADS

Bread is one of the things we truly love, and none of us really wanted any diet that made us give it up. So....

As regards turkey or buffalo burgers, Bonnie prefers hers without a bun, but William, and Bruce like one. While a regular, plain, white bun doesn't have too many calories, it, also, doesn't have much flavor; so, we've found that by using really good artesian bread, and splitting it lengthwise, then slicing into 2½-3" slices, we can make our own buns.

NOTE: If the bread is really thick, you can split it lengthways into three long sections, saving the middle for later, possibly to toast for breakfast.

NOTE: Another good tip is to make the Outside-In Burgers, from our *BACK OF THE BOAT GOURMET COOKING*, only cutting back on the amount of ingredients that you mix with the meat. By making these burgers with cheese, and other ingredients, mixed in with the meat, you can use less without giving up flavor (See Recipe under **FOWL**). Using ground turkey, or chicken, or buffalo, or even lean ground beef, leaving off the mayo or ranch dressing, a burger can be eaten while you diet. We tend to get into trouble, because we overindulge on the size of the burger (3 or 4 ounces is really the ideal portion), and because of all the things we pile on. And, of course, omit the macaroni and potato salad and have a green salad, grilled veggies, or even grilled fruit, instead (watermelon is delicious when grilled lightly, and it goes exceptionally well with grilled burgers).

Bread Sticks

These Bread Sticks satisfy our appetite for bread when we use them in place of a roll, or chunk of bread, to accompany our salad or soup.

Preheat oven to 400° (or use broiler or grill).

1 slice Diet Bread (40-45 calories per slice).

Spritz with extra virgin olive oil (1 spritz should do it).

Optional: rub with a garlic clove, or sprinkle with a dash of garlic powder, garlic salt, Italian seasoning, or cheese (Parmesan or Asiago).

Cut lengthways into 4 sections.

Bake at 400° until crisp and slightly toasted (if using grill or broiler, toast each side until brown and crisp).

Makes 2 servings.

About 20-22 calories (slightly more if using the cheese).

DESSERTS

Usually if we feel the need for dessert....

We have a piece of Xocai® healthy chocolate.

Or....

Fresh fruit, grilled, or drizzled with balsamic vinegar.

Then again....

Xocai® Chocolate Fondue
(Adapted from
***BACK OF THE BOAT GOURMET COOKING*)**

8 ounces of Xocai® Nuggets or X Power Squares
16 fresh long stemmed strawberries

Melt the chocolate in a bowl over hot, but not boiling, water until melted.

Transfer to a fondue pot on a platter and arrange the strawberries along side—or dip the strawberries in the chocolate and arrange on the platter.

Serve immediately.

Makes 4 servings.

250 calories a serving.

A bit of a calorie splurge, but, nevertheless, a healthy dessert.

WINES

We enjoy a glass of wine whenever our calorie allotments allow it…or we plan for it in our menu for the day.

Try mixing a half-and-half combination of Xocai® energy drink Xe® with inexpensive champagne.

We may not be as thin as we want to be, but we feel fabulous! All we can say is....

HELLO GORGEOUS!

HELLO HANDSOME!

RECIPE INDEX

Berry Vinaigrette, 102
Bleu-Cheese Dressing, 103
Bread Sticks, 156
BREADS, 155
Caesar Dressing, 104
Cauliflower Soup, 92
Crab-Quesadilla with Avocado, 127
DAIRY, 136
DESSERTS, 158
Dijon-Yogurt Dressing, 105
FISH AND SEAFOOD, 125
FOWL, 138
Gazpacho, 93
Green Bean Casserole—Bonnie-Style, 144
Grilled Tomato Tarts, 116
Honey-Mustard Dressing, 106
Honey-Pecan Crusted Chicken, 141
Inside-Out Turkey Burgers, 143
Lemon Sauce, 147
Lemony Herb Pasta, 152
Marinated Goat Cheese, 136
Onion Soup, 95

Onion Straws, 115
Oven-Roasted Garlic and Herb Potatoes, 120
PASTAS, 151
Pear Salad, 99
Poached Salmon with Orange Relish, 129
Potatoes, 119
Quick Berry Vinegar, 110
SALAD, 99
SALAD DRESSINGS, 101
Salmon with Berry Vinaigrette, 130
SAUCES, 147
Sole Stuffed with Crab, 133
Sole with White Wine and Grapes, 132
SOUPS, 92
Spice Rub, 126
Spinach Soufflés, 121
Steamed Vegetable Platter, 123
Sun-Dried Tomato and Sausage Pasta, 153
Tetrazzini (Chicken or Turkey), 144
Tortilla Soup, 96
Turkey (or Chicken) Gravy, 148
VEGETABLES, 111
VINEGAR, 109
Xocai® Chocolate Fondue, 158
Yogurt Cheese, 107
Yogurt-Mayonnaise Dressing, 107

ABOUT THE AUTHORS

BONNIE CLARK and husband Bruce were born, raised, met, and married in the Spokane, Washington, area, and have since raised their family there. Bonnie's interest in cooking started at a very early age when her Mother went to work, and Bonnie started planning and preparing dinners for the family. Her passion for cooking and entertaining grew, bolstered by her close connection and participation in her mother-in-law's professional catering business. Finally, enough family and friends told her she "should write a cookbook" that she decided, maybe, it was time she did. As it happens, her cousin, help- and cook-book author, William Maltese, fellow gourmand, wine connoisseur, and avid boater, was looking to do the same thing, and *BACK OF THE BOAT GOURMET COOKING* was born, followed by *EVEN GOURMANDS NEED TO DIET*. The latter contains some common-sense observations on dieting from two people daily subjected to good food, good wine, and the necessity to count calories.

Bonnie's Xocai® chocolate-for-sale site:

http://www.richesinchocolate.com

Check out her other website

http://www.facebook.com/backoftheboatgourmet-cooking

WILLIAM MALTESE, the author of his best-selling *WILLIAM MALTESE'S WINE TASTER'S DIARY: SPOKANE/PULLMAN WA*, and (along with A.B. Gayle) his *WILLIAM MALTESE'S WINE TASTER'S DIARY: IN SEARCH OF THE PERFECT G ON AUSTRALIA'S MORNINGTON PENINSULA*, and (along with Adrienne Z. Milligan) his *THE GLUTEN-FREE WAY: MY WAY*, and (along with Bonnie Clark) his *BACK OF THE BOAT GOURMET COOKING*, for "The Traveling Gourmand" imprint of Wildside/Borgo Press, was born in the Pacific Northwest, has a B.A. in Marketing/Advertising, and spent an honorable tour of duty in the U.S. Army where he achieved the rank of E-5. He started his career writing for men's pulp magazines, and has since had published more than 200 books, fiction and nonfiction, in every genre, while being honored with a listing in the prestigious Who's Who in America. For more information on William, pick up a copy of :

DRAQUALIAN SILK: A COLLECTOR'S AND BIBLIOGRAPHICAL GUIDE TO THE BOOKS OF WILLIAM MALTESE 1969-2010

http://www.wildsidebooks.com/Draqualian-Silk-A-Collectors-and-Bibliographical-Guide-to-the-Books-of-William-Maltese-1969-2010-by-William-Maltese-trade-pb_p_4908.html

William's Xocai® chocolate site:

http://www.mxi.myvoffice.com/williammaltese/

And check out his websites:

http://www.williammaltese.com

http://www.facebook.com/williammaltese

http://www.theglutenfreewaymyway.com/

http://www.facebook.com/backoftheboatgourmet-cooking

http://www.facebook.com/winetastersdiary

http://www.facebook.com/flickerwarriors

http://www.facebook.com/draqual

http://www.myspace.com/williammaltese

http://www.myspace.com/draqual

http://www.myspace.com/flickerwarriors

www.facebook.com/evengourmandshavetodiet

www.ingramcontent.com/pod-product-compliance
Lightning Source LLC
LaVergne TN
LVHW041624070426
835507LV00008B/431